Sirt food diet 2 in 1

Diet + cookbook

How you can start burn fat and active your "skinny gene" with tasty recipes.

BONUS: 4 weeks meal plan

Contents

SIRT Food Diet

The new step by step guide for beginners to start losing weight including meals plan, exercise and recipes

are for clarifying purposes only and are the owned by the owners themselves, not affiliated with this document.

Introduction

The Sirtfood Diet is a food lovers' diet. You cannot expect people to eat the way you do it for the long term. The Sirtfood Diet is turning all of that on its head.

The benefits are all from eating delicious food, and not from what you don't eat. The better food you consume, the greater the rewards you enjoy. It also encourages us to rekindle the lost relationships of enjoying mealtime. Whether it's being on a movie set, being on a music world tour, or managing a bustling home, the business you keep connecting with as a family, depends on what your daily life means. Meals are an event where all come together to enjoy the company of each other. That can be done easily with the Sirtfood Diet. Eat freely, without guilt. Knowing the food, you eat feeds on your wellbeing. The meal plans are realistic and easy to follow, while still delivering delicious meals. There's real satisfaction to see empty plates at the end of a meal and everyone is content. The word diet in this book's title can almost be a mishap. In the traditional sense this isn't a diet but a method of preparing for good. It's for anyone wanting to put their body in a healthier state and feel their best while still enjoying their life and food. It's for people who want to see big differences from small changes, and for those who want weight loss that can last without spending hours in the gym or starving. This book will change your mind set about a word' Diet' and it also covers all the questions that will come to your mind once you start reading it.

The sheer breadth of benefits experienced by people has been a revelation, all achieved by merely basing their diet on accessible and affordable foods that most people already enjoy eating. And that is all that the Sirtfood Diet needs. It's about extracting the advantages of daily products that we've always been meant to eat, but in the right quantities and formulations to give us the body composition and well-being that we all want so desperately, and that can finally change our lives.

It doesn't allow you to implement extreme calorie limits, nor does it involve grueling fitness regimens (although remaining generally active is a good thing, of course). And just a juicer is the only piece of equipment you'll require. However, unlike any other diet out there that focuses on what to eliminate, the Sirtfood Diet focuses on what to add.

I've experienced firsthand these astounding benefits, and so have my friends and family members. We've gone from saying we would never go on a diet to never eating any other way. Now it's your chance to experience and enjoy it too!

To sum it up, Sirtfood diet will help:

- To lose weight by burning fat but not muscles
- Burn fat from the stomach area
- Keep your body for long-term weight loss success
- To look and feel better
- Live a longer, healthier and perfect life

Chapter 1: Purpose of Sirtfood

What makes the Sirtfood Diet so powerful is their ability to switch to an ancient gene family that exists within each of us. The name for that gene family is sirtuin. Sirtuins are different as they orchestrate mechanisms deep inside our cells that involve things as essential as our capacity to burn fat, our sensitivity— or not — to disease, and eventually also our life span. The influence of sirtuins is so powerful that they are now referred to as "chief metabolic regulators." 1 Just what anyone who wishes to lose a few pounds and lead a long and healthy life would want to be in control.

Throughout recent years, sirtuins have, unsurprisingly, become the subject of intense scientific research. The first sirtuin was found in yeast back in 1984, and research only started in the course of the next three decades when it was reported that sirtuin activation enhances life span, first in yeast, and then up to mice. Why the excitement? Because the basic principles of cellular metabolism are almost identical from yeast to humans and everything in between. If you can manipulate something as tiny as budding yeast and see a benefit, then repeat it in higher organisms like mice, the potential for realizing the same interests in humans exists.

1.1 An Appetite for Fasting

That takes us to fast. Consistently, the lifelong restriction of food intake has been shown to extend the life expectancy of lower organisms and mammals. This extraordinary finding is the reason for the custom of caloric restriction among some individuals, where daily calorie consumption is lowered by about 20 to 30 percent, as well as its popularized offshoot, intermittent fasting, which has become a standard weight-loss method, made famous by the likes of the 5:2 diet, or Fast Method. While we're still looking for proof of improved survival for humans from these activities, there's confirmation of benefits for what we might term "health span"— chronic disease decreases, and fat starts to melt away.

But let's be real, no matter how significant the benefits, fasting week in, week out, is a grueling enterprise that most of us don't want to sign up for. Even if we do, most of us are not able to stick to this.

Besides this, there are risks to fasting, mainly if we practice it for a long time. We mentioned in the introduction the side effects of hunger, irritability, fatigue, muscle loss and slowdown in metabolism. Yet current fasting programs could also place us at risk of starvation, impacting our well-being due to a decreased intake of essential nutrients. Fasting systems are also entirely inappropriate for large proportions of the populace, such as infants, women during breastfeeding, and very likely older adults. Although fasting has clearly proven advantages, it's not the magic bullet we'd like it to be. It had to wonder, is this really the way God was meant to make us slim and healthy? There's certainly a better path out there.

Our breakthrough came when we discovered that our ancient sirtuin genes were activated by mediating the profound benefits of caloric restriction and fasting. It may be helpful to think of sirtuins as guards at the crossroads of energy status and survival to better understand this. There, what they do is react to pressures. If nutrition is in short supply, there is a rise in tension on our cells, just as we see in the caloric restriction. The sirtuins sensed this, which then switched on and transmitted a constellation of powerful signals that radically altered the behavior of cells. Sirtuins ramp up our metabolism, increase our muscle efficiency, switch on fat burning, decrease inflammation, and repair any damage in our cells. Sirtuins, in turn, make us better, leaner, and safer.

1.2 An Energy for Exercise

It's not just caloric restriction and fasting that activates sirtuins; exercise does too. Sirtuins orchestrate the profound benefits of exercise just as they do in fasting. Yet while we are urged to participate in routine, moderate exercise for its multitude of advantages, it is not the method by which we are expected to focus our efforts on weight-loss. Research shows that the human body has developed ways of adapting spontaneously and reducing the amount of energy that we spend while exercising, seven implying that in order for exercise to be a successful weight-loss strategy, we need to devote considerable time and effort. The grueling fitness plans are the way Nature intended us to maintain a healthy weight is even more questionable in the light of studies now showing that too much activity can be harmful— weakening our immune systems, harming the liver, and leading to an early death.

So far, we have discovered that the key to activating our sirtuin genes is if we want to lose weight and be healthy. Up until now, diet and meditation have been the two proven ways to achieve this.

Unfortunately, the amounts needed for successful weight loss come with their drawbacks, and for most of us, this is simply incompatible with how we live twenty-first century lives. Luckily, there is a newly discovered, ground-breaking way to activate our sirtuin genes in the best way possible: sirtfood. As we will know early, these are the wonderful foods which are especially rich in specific natural plant chemicals, which have the ability to communicate to our sirtuin genes and turn them on. Essentially, they mimic the results of diet and exercise, which offer impressive advantages by burning fat in doing so., muscle building, and health-boosting that were previously unattainable.

SUMMARY

- Each one of us has an ancient gene family called sirtuins.

- Master metabolic regulators are sirtuins that regulate our ability to burn fat and maintain a healthy state.

- Sirtuins serve as energy sensors inside our cells and are triggered upon identification of energy shortages.

- Both fasts and exercises activate our sirtuin genes but can be challenging to adhere to and may even have drawbacks.

- You will replicate the results of fasting and exercise by eating a diet high in Sirtfoods and create the body you like.

Chapter 2: Masters of Muscles

One surprising result from our pilot trial that puzzled us was that the participants' muscle mass did not drop; instead, it rose by just over 1 pound on average. While it was common to see weight loss on the scales of 7 pounds, we saw something fascinating happening too. The injuries on the levels initially appeared more disappointing than this for almost two-thirds of our participants, though still very impressive, with a weight loss of just over 5 pounds. But when tests were done on body composition, we were astonished. In these participants, muscle mass was not only maintained; it had increased. The total muscle benefit for this category was almost 2 pounds, adding 7 pounds to what is called a "muscle gain-based weight loss."

This was totally unexpected and in stark contrast to what is typically the case for diets for weight loss, where people lose some fat but also lose muscle. For any diet which limits calories, it's the classic trade-off: you kiss good-bye muscle as well as fat. This is not at all surprising when you consider that cells change from growth mode to survival mode as we rob the body of nutrition and will use the protein from the muscle as food.

2.1 What's Good about maintaining Muscles?

So, what's that big deal? Do you know? Firstly, that means you're going to look much better. Stripping away weight while maintaining muscle leads to a healthy, toned, and competitive body that is more attractive. And more specifically, you should remain good looking. The skeletal muscle is the main factor that accounts for the daily energy output of our body, which ensures the more muscle that you have, the more calories that you use, even when you rest. This helps support further weight loss and increases the likelihood of long-term success. As we now learn, weight loss with typical diet results from both fat loss and muscle loss, and thereby we see a marked decline in the metabolic rate. This induces the body to regain weight once more regular eating habits are resumed. But you burn more fat with a minimal drop in metabolic rate by holding your muscle mass with Sirtfoods. This provides the perfect basis for weight-loss success over the long term.

In addition, muscle mass and function are predictors of well-being and healthy aging, and maintaining the muscle prevents the development of chronic diseases such as diabetes and osteoporosis, as well as keeping us mobile into older age. Importantly, it also seems to make us happy, with scientists believing that even the way sirtuins retain muscle has implications for stress-related disorders, including depression reduction.

All in all, weight loss when maintaining the body is a biggie and an even more desirable outcome. It's a unique feature of the Sirtfood Diet, and we need to get back to the sirtuins, so their substantial impact on the muscle to better understand why.

2.2 Sirtuins and Muscles Mass

In the body, there is a family of genes that function as guardians of our muscle and, when under stress, avoid its breakdown: the sirtuins. SIRT is a potent Muscle Breakdown Inhibitor. As long as SIRT is activated, even when we are fasting, muscle breakdown is prevented, and we continue to burn fat for fuel.

But SIRT's benefits aren't ending with preserving muscle mass. The sirtuins work to increase our skeletal muscle mass. We need to delve into the exciting world of stem cells and illustrate how that process functions. Our muscle comprises a particular type of stem cell, which is called a satellite cell that regulates its development and regeneration. Satellite cells just sit there quietly most of the time, but they are activated when a muscle gets damaged or stressed. By things like weight training, this is how our muscles grow stronger. SIRT is essential for activating satellite cells, and without its activity, muscles are significantly smaller because they no longer have the capacity to develop or regenerate properly.6 However, by increasing SIRT activity, we give a boost to our satellite cells, which encourages muscle growth and recovery.

2.3 SirtFood Versus Fasting

This leads to a big question: if activation of the sirtuin increases muscle mass, why do we lose muscle when we fast? Fasting also stimulates our sirtuin genes, after all. And therein is one of fasting's big pitfalls.

Stay with us as we dig into the mechanics of this. Not all skeletal muscles are created equal to each other. We have two main types, named type-1 and type-2, conveniently. Type-1 tissue is used for movements of longer duration, while the type-2 muscle is used for short bursts of more intense activity. And here's where it gets intriguing: fasting only increases SIRT activity in type-1 muscle fibers, not type-2, So type-1 muscle fiber size is maintained and even noticeably increases when we fast. Sadly, in complete contrast to what happens in type-1 fibers during fasting, SIRT rapidly decreases in type-2 fibers. This means that fat burning slows down, and muscle breaks down to provide fuel, instead.

But fasting for the muscles is a double-edged sword, with our type-2 fibers taking a hit. Type-2 fibers form the bulk of our concept of muscle. So even though our type-1 fiber mass is growing, with fasting, we still see a substantial overall loss of muscle. If we were able to stop the breakup, it would not only make us look aesthetically healthy but also help to promote more loss of weight. And the way to do this is to combat the decrease in SIRT in muscle fiber type-2 that is caused by fasting.

Researchers at Harvard Medical School tested this in an elegant mice study. They showed that the signals for muscle breakdown were switched off by stimulating SIRT activity in type-2 fibers during fasting, and no muscle loss occurred. The researchers then went to one step forward and checked the effects of increased SIRT behavior on the muscle while feeding the mice instead of fasted, and found it triggered a very rapid growth of the muscle.

Within a week, muscle fibers with increased levels of SIRT activity showed an amazing weight gain of 20 percent.

These findings are very similar to the outcome of our Sirtfood Diet trial, though, in effect, our study has been milder. By increasing SIRT activity by eating a diet rich in sirtfoods, most participants had no muscle loss— and for many, it was only a moderate fast, muscle mass that increased.

2.4 Keeping Muscles Young

And that is not just the thickness of the body. SIRT's prolific effects on the muscle extend to the way it works too. As the muscle ages, it loses the ability to activate SIRT. This makes it less sensitive to exercise benefits and more vulnerable to free radicals and inflammation destruction, resulting in what is known as oxidative stress. Gradually muscles wither, become softer, and fatigue faster. But if we can increase SIRT activation, we can stop the decline associated with aging.

Indeed, by activating SIRT to stop the loss of muscle mass and function we usually see with aging, we see multiple related health benefits, including the halting of bone loss and prevention of increased chronic systemic inflammation (known as inflamaging), as well as improvements in mobility and overall quality of life. So, interestingly, the latest research indicates that the higher the polyphenol level (and thus sirtuin-activating nutrients) in older people's diets, the higher the security they enjoy against deteriorating physical performance with age.

Don't be fooled into thinking that those incentives extend only to the elderly, far from that. By the age of twenty-five, the signs of aging will begin, and the muscle gradually erodes, with 10 percent loss of muscle around age forty (although overall weight tends to increase) and a loss of 40 percent by age seventy. Yet there is growing evidence that the activation of our sirtuin genes will inhibit and reverse all of this.

Loss of muscle, development, and function: sirtuin behavior plays a crucial role in all of this. Stack it up, and it's no surprise that sirtuins were identified as master regulators of muscle growth in a recent review in the prestigious medical journal Nature, with growing sirtuin activation cited as one of the promising new avenues for combating muscle loss, thereby increasing the quality of life, as well as reducing disease and death.

Looking at the powerful effects our sirtuin genes can have on the muscles, our pilot trial's shock results no longer seemed so shocking. We started to realize that driving weight loss when feeding our muscles was achievable through a diet rich in Sirtfood.

But it's just the beginning. In the next chapter, we'll see Sirtfoods' benefits extending so much further, to all aspects of health and quality of life.

SUMMARY

- Amid weight loss, we found that people either retained or even gained muscle through the Sirtfood diet. This is because the sirtuins are chief muscle regulators.

- By activating sirtuins, muscle breakdown can be both prevented and muscle regeneration promoted.

- Triggering SIRT will help prevent the progressive muscle loss that we see with age.

- Activating your sirtuin genes will not only make you look leaner but will also help you stay healthier and function better as you age.

Chapter 3: Fighting Fat

One of the surprising results from our Sirtfood Diet pilot study wasn't just how much weight the participants lost, which was unusual enough— it was the amount of weight loss that fascinated us. What attracted our eye was the fact that a lot of people lost weight without missing any muscle. In reality, watching people gain muscle wasn't rare.

It left us with an inevitable conclusion: fat had merely melted away.

Achieving a substantial fat loss requires typically a tremendous effort, either significantly decreasing calories or participating in extraordinary exercise levels or both. Yet counter to that, our participants either retained or reduced their level of exercise and did not even report feel particularly hungry. In reality, some also refused to consume all of the food they had been supplied with.

Why is it even that possible? It is only when we understand what happens to our fat cells when there is elevated sirtuin production that we can begin to make sense of these remarkable results.

Mice that have been genetically engineered to have elevated SIRT rates are leaner and more metabolically involved, the sirtuin gene that causes fat loss. In comparison, mice who lack SIRT are more overweight and have more metabolic diseases. If we look at individuals, SIRT levels in obese people's body fat were found to be markedly lower than their healthy-weight equivalents. Those with elevated SIRT gene expression, on the other side, become leaner and more immune to weight gain. Scale all that together, and you begin to get a picture of how critical sirtuins are to decide how we stay lean or get overweight, and why you can produce these amazing results by increasing sirtuin activity. This is because we get advantages on multiple levels by sirtuins, beginning at the very heart of everything: the genes that regulate weight gain. To grasp this further, we need to delve deeper into what is occurring in our bodies, which is allowing us to gain some weight.

3.1 Busting Fat

We'll clarify this in terms of a drug-ring film in Hollywood. The streets flooded with narcotics is our body overflowing with fat. The drug pushers on the street corners are the source of the weight gain peddling responses in our heads.

But in fact, it's just the low-level losers. The real villain is behind it all, masterminding the entire operation, guiding any transaction that the peddlers make. This antagonist is referred to in our film as PPAR-π (peroxisome proliferator-activated receptor-ÿ). PPAR-ÿ orchestrates the mechanism of fat gain by clicking on the genes required to start synthesizing and storing fat. You will slash supply to avoid the accumulation of fat. Start PPAR-ÿ and you start fat gain successfully.

Meet our hero SIRT, who rises to push the enemy down. With the thief locked up safely, there's no one to pull strings, and the whole fat-gain enterprise crumbles. With PPAR-π's operation stopped, SIRT is turning its focus to "cleaning the streets." Not only is this achieved by shutting down fat development and storage, as we have seen, but it is changing our metabolism so that we continue to rid the body of excess fat. Like every successful crime-fighting character, SIRT has a sidekick, identified as PGC-1α, a central receptor in our cells. It actively encourages the formation of what is known as mitochondria. These are the tiny factories of energy that live inside each of our cells— they drive the body. The more we have the mitochondria, the more we can generate the oil. But as well as encouraging more mitochondria, PGC-1α also urges them to burn fat as the fuel of choice to make the electricity. So fat accumulation is prevented on the one side, and fat burning on the other decreases.

3.2 WAT OR BAT?

We have looked so far at the impact of SIRT on fat loss on a well-known fat type called white adipose tissue (WAT). This is the type of fat that weight gain coincides with. This specializes in preservation and growth, is persistent, and secretes a variety of inflammatory chemicals that prevent fat burning and promote more accumulation of fat, leaving us overweight and obese. That's why weight gain always begins gradually but can escalate so quickly.

But the sirtuin tale has another interesting twist, including a lesser-known type of fat, brown adipose tissue (BAT), which acts very differently. BAT is advantageous to us in complete contrast to white adipose tissue and needs to get used up. Brown adipose tissue helps us expend energy and has developed into mammals to allow them to dissipate large amounts of heat-shaped fat. This is regarded as a thermogenic influence and is essential to helping small mammals thrive in cold temperatures. Babies often contain considerable amounts of brown adipose tissue in humans, although it declines shortly after birth, leaving smaller amounts in adults.

This is where the activation of SIRT is doing something truly amazing. It turns on genes in our white adipose tissue so that it morphs and absorbs the characteristics of brown adipose tissue in what is considered a "browning effect." This suggests that our fat stores tend to function in a completely different way— instead of storing energy, they start mobilizing it for disposal. Sirtuin stimulation, as we can see, has an effective direct action on fat cells, allowing the fat to melt away. But there, it's not over.

The sirtuins also have a positive influence on the most critical weight control hormones. Activation of the sirtuin increases insulin production. It helps to reduce the insulin resistance— the failure of our cells to react to insulin adequately— which is heavily involved in weight gain. SIRT also stimulates our thyroid hormones ' release and operation, which play several standard functions in improving our metabolism and eventually, the pace we burn fat at.

3.3 Appetite Control

There was one aspect we couldn't get our minds around in our pilot study: the people didn't get hungry given a drop-in calorie. In reality, several people struggled to consume all of the food that was offered.

One of the significant advantages of the Sirtfood Diet is that without the need for a long-term calorie restriction, we can achieve great benefits. The very first week of diet is the process of hyper-success, where we pair mild fasting with an excess of strong Sirtfoods for a double blow to weight. So, we predicted sure signs of hunger here, as with all of the fasting regimens. But we've had virtually zero!

We found the answer, as we trawled through analysis. It's all thanks to the body's primary appetite-regulating hormone, leptin, called the "satiety hormone." As we feed, leptin decreases, signaling the hypothalamus inhibiting desire to a part of the brain. Conversely, leptin signaling to the mind declines as we fly, which makes us feel thirsty.

Leptin is so effective in controlling appetite that early expectations where it could be treated as a "magic bullet" for combating obesity. But that vision was broken by the fact that the metabolic disorder found in obesity causes leptin to avoid correctly functioning. Through obesity, the volume of leptin that can reach the brain is not only decreased, but the hypothalamus also becomes desensitized to its behavior. This is regarded as leptin resistance: there is leptin, but it doesn't work correctly anymore. Therefore, for many overweight individuals, the brain continues to think they are underfed even though they consume plenty, which triggers for them to continue to seek calories.

The consequence of this is that while the amount of leptin in the blood is necessary to control appetite, how much of it enters the brain and can have an effect on the hypothalamus is far more relevant. It is here that the Sirtfoods shine.

New evidence indicates that the nutrients present in Sirtfoods have unique advantages in overcoming leptin resistance. This is by both increasing leptin delivery to the brain and through the hypothalamus ' response to leptin behavior.

Going back to our original question: Why don't the Sirtfood Diet make people feel hungry? Given a decrease in blood leptin rates during the mild quick, which would usually raise motivation, incorporating Sirtfoods into the diet makes leptin signals more productive, leading to better control of appetite.

As we'll see later, Sirtfoods also has powerful effects on our taste centers, meaning we get a lot more pleasure and satisfaction from our food and therefore don't fall into the overeating trap to feel happy.

Sirtuins are expected to be a brand-new concept for even the most committed dietitians. But hitting the sirtuins, our metabolism's master regulators, is the foundation of any effective diet for weight loss. Tragically, the very existence of our modern society, with abundant food and sedentary lifestyles, creates a perfect storm to shut down our sirtuin operation, and we see all around us the effects of this.

The good thing is that we know what sirtuins are, how fat accumulation is managed, and how fat burning is encouraged, and most significantly, how to turn them on. And with this revolutionary breakthrough, the key to successful and lasting weight loss is now yours to bear.

SUMMARY

- Fat on Sirtfood Diet melts away. This is because sirtuins have the power to determine whether we stay thin or are getting fat.

- Activating SIRT inhibits PPAR-π, thereby preventing fat development and storage.

- Interestingly, triggering SIRT switches on PGC-1α, which allows our cells more fuel producers and enhances fat burning.

- On the Sirtfood Diet, you are unlikely to feel hungry because it tends to control the hunger in your brain.

Chapter 4: Well-Being Wonders

Society is getting fatter and sicker given all the incredible advances in modern medicine—70 percent of all fatalities are due to chronic illness, a truly shocking figure. Radical, and immediate, change is needed.

And as we've seen, all of this can begin to change. We will burn fat by stimulating our ancient sirtuin genes and create a leaner, stronger body. And with sirtuins at the center of our metabolism, our physiology master engineers, their significance reaches far beyond the structure of the body itself, to every aspect of our well-being.

4.1 What are Sirt Foods?

When we cut back on calories, this creates an energy shortage that activates what is known as the "skinny gene," triggering a raft of positive change. It puts the body in a kind of survival mode where fat is stopped from being stored, and healthy growth processes are put on hold. Alternatively, the body is shifting its focus to burning up its fat stores and putting on active housekeeping genes that rebuild and rejuvenate our cells, effectively giving them a spring clean. The upshot is weight loss and heightened disease resistance. But cutting calories, as many dieters know, comes at a cost.

Reducing energy consumption in the short term induces nausea, irritability, exhaustion, and lack of muscle. Long-term restriction on calories is causing our metabolism to stagnate. This is the collapse of all calorie-restrictive diets and paves the way for a piling back on the weight. For these reasons, 99 percent of dietitians are doomed to long-term failure.

All of this has prompted us to pose a big question: is it feasible to trigger our slim gene with all the great benefits they come and all those disadvantages without having to stick to an extreme calorie restriction?

Sirtfoods are especially rich in particular nutrients that can activate the same skinny genes in our bodies when we consume them as calorie restriction does. Those genes are called sirtuins. They first appeared in a landmark study in 2003, when researchers found resveratrol, a compound found in red-grape skin and red-wine, dramatically increased the lifetime of the petals. Incredibly, resveratrol had the same effect as calorie restriction on longevity, but this was achieved without reducing the energy intake. Studies have since shown that resveratrol has the potential to extend life in worms, fish, and even honeybees. Early-stage experiments from mice to humans indicate that resveratrol protects from the harmful effects of high-calorie, high-fat, and high-sugar diets; promotes healthy ageing by slowing age-related diseases and improves mobility. Essentially, the results of calorie restriction and activity have been proven to be imitation.

Red wine was dubbed as the first Sirtfood with its rich resveratrol material, describing the health benefits associated with its intake, and even why people who drink red wine get less weight. That is just the beginning of the Sirtfood tale, however.

The world of health research was at the cusp of something big with the discovery of resveratrol, and the pharmaceutical industry wasted no time jumping on board. Researchers have begun screening thousands of different chemicals for their capacity to activate our sirtuin genes. That revealed a number of natural plant compounds with significant sirtuin-activating properties, not just resveratrol. It was also found that a given food could contain a whole spectrum of these plant compounds, which could work together to both aid absorption and maximize the sirtuin-activating effect of that food. This had been one of the great resveratrol puzzles. Resveratrol experimenting scientists often needed to use far higher doses than we know when consumed as part of the red wine to provide a benefit. Nevertheless, unlike resveratrol, red wine contains a variety of other natural compounds for plants, including high amounts of piceatannol and quercetin, myricetin and epicatechin, each of which has been shown to activate our sirtuin genes individually and, more importantly, to function in combination. The dilemma for the pharmaceutical industry is that the next major breakthrough product cannot be sold as a vitamin or food category. So instead, they spent hundreds of millions of dollars in the expectation of uncovering a Shangri-la pill to create and conduct tests of organic compounds. Multiple studies of sirtuin-activating drugs for a multitude of chronic diseases are currently underway, and the first FDA-approved study to examine whether the drug would slow down ageing.

If we have learnt anything from history, it's that we shouldn't hold much hope for this pharmaceutical ambrosia, as tantalizing as that may seem. The medicine and wellness companies have continuously tried to emulate the effects of products and lifestyles by single supplements and medications.

And it has come up short again and again. Why wait ten more years for these so-called miracle medications to be approved, and the potential side effects they offer, because right now we have all the incredible benefits accessible through the food we eat at our fingertips?

So, while the pharmaceutical industry is chasing a drug-like magic bullet aggressively, we need to retrain our attention to dieting. At the same time, those efforts were underway, the landscape of nutritional research was also shifting, raising some big questions of its own. Red wine, on the one hand, were there other high-level foods of these different nutrients able to trigger our sirtuin genes? And if so, what effects did they have on triggering fat loss and combating disease?

4.2 All Fruits and Vegetables Are Not Created Equally

Researchers at Harvard University have conducted two of the most significant nutritional studies in US history since 1986: The Health Professionals Follow-Up Study, which examines men's dietary habits and health, and the Nurses' Health Study, which investigates the same for women. Building on this vast wealth of data, researchers explored the link between more than 124,000 people's dietary habits and changes in body weight over a twenty-four-year period ending in 2011.

They found something striking. Eating some plant foods staved off weight gain as part of a standard American diet, but eating others had no impact whatsoever. What were they different from each other? It all boiled down to whether there were different kinds of natural plant chemicals such as polyphenols that made the food beautiful. Almost all of us tend to put on weight when we mature, but the intake of higher quantities of polyphenols had a notable impact on avoiding this. Only certain types of polyphenols stood out when examined in greater detail as being useful in keeping people slim, the researchers found. The same groups of natural plant chemicals that the pharmaceutical industry was furiously trying to turn into a wonder pill for their ability to turn on our sirtuin genes were among those users.

The result was profound: When it comes to controlling our weight, not all plant foods (including fruits and vegetables) are equivalent. Alternatively, we need to start researching plant foods for their polyphenol material and then examine their ability to switch on our "skinny" sirtuin genes.

This is a radical idea that goes against the prevailing orthodoxy of our times. It's time to let go of the general blanket recommendations as part of a balanced diet that asks us to eat two cups of fruit and two and a half cups of vegetables a day. We only need to glance around to see how far that has had effects.

Something else became apparent with this shift in judging how plant foods are good for us. The many foods that supposedly health experts warned us off, such as chocolate, coffee, and tea, are so rich in sirtuin-activating polyphenols that they trump most fruits and vegetables out there. How many days are we grimacing when we chew our veggies because we are advised that this is the right thing to do, only to feel guilty if we even look at the sweet cookie during dinner? The ultimate irony is that cacao is one of the best foods that we might be consuming. The intake has now been shown to activate sirtuin genes, with multiple benefits for regulating body weight by burning fat, reducing appetite, and increasing muscle function. And that is before we take its multitude of other health benefits into account, more of which will come later.

In all, we have established twenty polyphenol-rich foods that have been shown to activate our sirtuin genes, and together these form the basis of the Sirtfood Diet. While the story began as the initial Sirtfood with red wine, we now know that these other nineteen foods equal or beat it for their sirtuin-activating polyphenol content. In addition to chocolate, these include other well-known and delicious products such as extra virgin olive oil, red onions, garlic, parsley, chilies, broccoli, bananas, walnuts, capers, bacon, green tea, and even coffee. While each food has impressive health credentials of its own, as we are about to see, when we combine these foods to make a whole diet, the real magic happens.

4.3 A Common Link Among all Other Diets

When we further researched, we learned that the most substantial concentrations of sirtfoods were contained in the diets of those with the lowest disease and obesity rates in the world — from the Kuna American Indians, who are resistant to high blood pressure and exhibit remarkably low rates of obesity, diabetes, cancer, and early death, thanks to a fantastically rich consumption of Sirtfood cocoa; to Okinawa, Japan.

But it's the diet that is the envy of the rest of the Western world, a traditional Mediterranean diet, where Sirtfoods stands out for its benefits. Obesity simply does not prevail here, and the exception is a chronic illness, not the norm. Extra virgin olive oil, wild leafy greens, almonds, fruit, red wine, seeds, and spices are all-powerful syrups, both appearing prominently in Mediterranean natural diets. Given the recent consensus that following a Mediterranean diet is more effective than counting calories for weight loss, and more effective than pharmaceutical drugs to stop the disease, the scientific world has been left in awe.

It takes us to the 2013 release of PREDIMED, a game-changing analysis of the Mediterranean Diet. It was performed on about 7,400 people at high risk of cardiovascular disease, and the results were positive that the study was effectively stopped early—after just five years. PREDIMED's premise was gorgeously simple. This asked what the difference between a Mediterranean-style diet augmented by either extra virgin olive oil or nuts (especially walnuts) and a more traditional modern-day diet would be. And what a difference.

The dietary change reduced the incidence of cardiovascular disease by about 30 percent, so drug companies can only dream of a result. With further follow-up, a 30 percent decrease in diabetes was also observed, along with significant drops in inflammation, changes in memory and brain health, and a massive 40 percent reduction in obesity, with substantial fat loss, particularly around the stomach area.

Yet researchers were initially unable to explain what these dramatic benefits produced. Neither the amounts of calories, fats, and sugars are eaten— the standard measures used to evaluate the food we eat— nor the levels of physical activity differentiated between the groups to explain the results. Something else had to get going.

The eureka moment then happened. Both extra virgin olive oil and walnuts are notable for their exceptional sirtuin-activating polyphenols content. Mostly, by adding these to a healthy Mediterranean diet in significant amounts, what the researchers unwittingly created was a super-rich Sirtfood diet, and they found it delivered terrific results.

So PREDIMED-analyzing researchers came up with a smart hypothesis. Unless actually, it is the polyphenols that count, they mused, then those who eat more of them would reap their combined benefits by living the longest. So, they were running the statistics, and the results were staggering. Those who consumed the highest polyphenol levels had 37 percent fewer deaths over just five years compared to those who ate the lowest. Intriguingly, this is double the mortality reduction that treatment with the most commonly prescribed blockbuster statin drugs is found to bring. Eventually, we had the reason for the mind-blowing benefits found in this test, and it was more effective than any existing drug.

The researchers also noticed something else unusual.

Although historically several studies have found that individual Sirtfoods impart remarkable health benefits, they have never been comprehensive enough to extend life potentially. The first such was PREDIMED. The difference was that they were looking at a food pattern rather than a single food. Different foods provide different polyphenols that activate sirtuin, which work in harmony to produce a much more powerful result than any single food can. This has left an irrepressible conclusion for us. Real wellness is not captured by a single nutrient or even a "wonderful meal." What you need is a full diet packed with a mix of synergistic Sirtfoods that all function. And that is what led to Sirtfood Diet being developed.

4.4 The Sirt Foods Empirical Study

Bit by bit, we've compiled all the observations from traditional cultures and the findings from major scientific studies, culminating in PREDIMED, one of the best dietary studies ever. But even PREDIMED's results came through chance as did many health breakthroughs. It never started to formulate and check a Sirtfood diet. Only later did science discover that this was indeed what PREDIMED had done.

This meant that the diet had not included many Sirtfoods that could have further increased its immense benefits.

In addition, all the research to date had identified the benefits for long-term weight management and disease reduction.

But we still didn't know how easily such effects could be recognized for body weight and well-being. We all want to protect our health in the future, but don't we want to look and feel right here and now?

To answer these questions, we wanted an experiment intentionally performed by the Sirtfood Diet that included all twenty of the most efficient SirtFoods with which we could collect earlier results measurements. So, we embarked on our pilot study.

Nestled in the middle of London, England, KX is one of the most coveted health and fitness facilities in Europe. That makes KX the perfect place to check the Sirtfood Diet's results is that it has its kitchen, which has provided us the chance not only to devise the diet but to bring it to life and evaluate it on the participants of the fitness center.

Our competences were obvious. Members would observe our built Sirtfood Diet for seven days in a row, and we would track their progress closely from start to finish, not only tracking their weight but also observing improvements in their body composition, which included testing how the diet influenced the fat and muscle levels in the body. Later, we added metabolic measures to see the diet's effects on blood sugar levels (glucose) and fats (such as triglycerides and cholesterol).

The first three days have been the most intense, with food intake limited to 1,000 calories a day. This is like a mild quick, which is necessary because the lower consumption of energy turns down signs of growth in the body and allows it to start clearing out old garbage from cells (a process known as autophagy) and kick-start fat burning. But unlike traditional fasting diets, this fast was gentle and short-lived, rendering it much more manageable, as shown by the exceptionally high adherence rate of 97.5 percent of the sample. We wanted to investigate the variations that were created by applying Sirtfoods to the usual drop associated with fasting diets. And they have been intense, as we were soon to find out.

Our primary objective was to make a big difference to the fat-burning results of this moderate calorie restriction by loading the Sirtfoods complete diet. This was done by basing the daily menu on three green beverages rich in Sirtfood, and one meal rich in Sirtfood.

At KX, calories were increased to 1,500 per day for the remaining four days of our study. Effectively this was only a rather small calorie deficit, but it turned down, and fat-burning signals turned up enough to hold development signals. Importantly, there was a jam-packed 1,500-calorie diet of Sirtfoods, comprising of two Sirtfood-rich green juices and two Sirtfood-rich meals per day.

4.5 The Results

The Sirtfood Diet was tested by forty, and thirty-nine members completed it at KX. Of those thirty-nine, two were obese in the trial, fifteen of them were overweight, and twenty-two had a healthy body mass index (BMI). The study was divided fairly even in gender, with twenty-one women and eighteen men. As participants of a health club, they were more inclined than the general population to participate and be conscious of healthy eating when they began.

The secret of many diets is to use a highly overweight and unhealthy sample of people to show the benefits, since at first, they lose weight the most and most drastically, effectively fluffing up the diet performance. Our rationale was the opposite: if with this relatively healthy population, we received good results, it would set the minimum benchmark of what could be accomplished.

The performance well exceeded our expectations, even healthy. The findings were clear and fantastic: an average weight reduction of 7 pounds in seven days after muscle growth is accounted for.

As if that wasn't inspiring enough, we've seen something else even more remarkable, which was the weight loss kind.

Typically, when people lose weight, they're going to lose some fat, but they're also going to lose some muscle— this is par for the diet course. We were amazed to discover the reverse. Our participants either kept their flesh or gained muscle. This is an infinitely more favorable type of weight loss, and a unique feature of the Sirtfood Diet, as we will find out later in the book.

No researcher struggled to see body composition changes. Yet note, without food deprivation or grueling fitness regimens, all this was done.

Here's what we found from our study

- Participants obtained spectacular and fast performance, dropping 7 pounds on average in seven days.

- Weight loss around the abdominal area was most noticeable.

- Muscle mass was either preserved or raised, rather than reduced.

- Rarely did the participants feel hungry.

- Participants felt a feeling of increased vitality and well-being.

- Participants reported having a better and healthier appearance.

4.6 Suirtins and The 70 Percent

Think of a condition you link with getting older and the likelihood of causing a loss of sirtuin involvement in the body. Sirtuin activation, for example, is excellent for heart health, protecting the muscle cells in the heart, and generally helping the heart muscle function better.[1] It also improves how our arteries work, helps us handle cholesterol more effectively, and protects against blockage of our arteries known as atherosclerosis.

As for diabetes? Activation of the sirtuin increases the amount of insulin that can be secreted and helps the bodywork more effectively. As it happens, metformin, one of the most common anti-diabetes medications, depends on SIRT for its beneficial effect.

Indeed, one pharmaceutical company is currently investigating the addition of natural sirtuin activators to diabetic metformin treatment, with results from animal studies showing a staggering 83% reduction in metformin dose required for the same effects.

As for the brain, sirtuins are again involved, with sirtuin activity found to be lower in patients with Alzheimer's. By contrast, activation of the sirtuin improves communication signals in the brain, enhances cognitive function, and reduces inflammation of the brain. This stops the accumulation of amyloid-β production and tau protein aggregation, two of the main damaging things we see happening in the brains of patients with Alzheimer's.

The next one is the teeth. Osteoblasts are a specific type of cell which is responsible for building new bone in our bodies. The more osteoblasts we get, the stronger our bones become. Activation of sirtuin not only stimulates the growth of osteoblast cells but also improves their survival. It allows the activation of sirtuin necessary for the protection of lifelong bones.

For sirtuin research, cancer has been a more controversial area. While a recent study shows that sirtuin activation helps suppress cancer tumors, scientists are only beginning to unravel this complex field. While there are so many other things to learn about this particular topic, as we shall see soon, those cultures that eat the most Sirtfoods have the lowest cancer rates.

Heart disease, arthritis, depression, osteoporosis, and most definitely cancer: this is an impressive list of diseases that can be avoided by sirtuin activation. It may come as no surprise to find out that cultures that already eat plenty of Sirtfoods as part of their traditional diets are experiencing longevity and well-being than most of us can hardly imagine, which you will hear more about very soon.

This leaves us with an exciting conclusion: only by adding the strongest sirtfoods in the world to your diet and having it a lifetime routine, you too can achieve this degree of well-being — and more — while you get the science you like.

SUMMARY

- For all the advances in modern science, we are getting fatter as a community.

- Seventy percent of all deaths are caused by chronic disease, with the vast majority having low sirtuin activity involved.

- Through triggering sirtuins, you can eliminate or forestall the Western world's most significant chronic diseases.

- By packing your diet full of Sirtfoods, you, too, can enjoy the same level of well-being as the healthiest and longest-living populations on the planet.

Chapter: 5 Sirt Foods

We've learned so far that sirtuins are an ancient gene family with the ability to help us burn fat, build muscle, and keep us super happy. It is well known that by caloric restriction, fasting, and exercise, sirtuins can be turned on, but there is another innovative way to achieve this: diet. We refer to the most active foods to activate sirtuins as Sirtfoods.

To understand the benefits of Sirtfoods, we need to learn about foods like fruits and vegetables very differently, and why they are perfect for us. Despite tons of evidence demonstrating that diets high in fruits, vegetables, and plant foods usually cut the risk of many chronic diseases, including the biggest killers, heart disease, and cancer, there is absolutely no doubt they do. This has been put down to their rich nutrient content, such as vitamins, minerals, and, of course, antioxidants, which is probably the greatest wellness buzzword of the last decade. But this is a very different story we are here to share.

The explanation Sirtfoods is so fantastic for you has nothing to do with the nutrients that we all know so well and hear about so much. Yes, they're all valuable things you need to get out of your diet, but with Sirtfoods there's something entirely different, and very unique. In reality, what if we turned that whole way of thinking on its ear and said that the explanation Sirtfoods is right for you is not that they nourish the body with essential nutrients, or provide antioxidants to mop up the damaging effects of free radicals, but quite the opposite: because they are full of weak toxins? This might sound crazy in an environment where almost every alleged "healthy food" is aggressively marketed focused on its antioxidant content. But it's a revolutionary idea, and one worth taking on.

5.1 What makes you stronger

Let's get back for a moment to the proven methods of triggering sirtuins: fasting and exercise. Evidence has shown consistently, as we have seen, that the allocation of dietary resources has significant effects for weight loss, wellbeing, and, quite likely, lifespan. Then there is fitness, with its numerous advantages for both body and mind, pointed out by the discovery that regular exercise slashes mortality rates dramatically. But what is the one thing they have in common?

The answer lies in: heat. All fasting and exercise cause the body to experience moderate stress that helps it to adjust by becoming stronger, more productive, and more durable. It is the reaction of the body to these slightly unpleasant stimuli— its adaptation— that, in the long run, should make us better, safer, and leaner. So, as we now learn, sirtuins orchestrate these highly beneficial modifications, which are turned on in the presence of these stressors, so spark a series of desirable changes in the body.

The technical term used to respond to those pressures is hormesis. It's the theory that if subjected to a low dose of a drug or stimulus that is otherwise harmful or fatal if administered at higher doses, you get a beneficial effect. Perhaps "things that don't kill you make you stronger," if you like. And that's just how fasting because exercising function. Hunger is fatal, so excessive exercise is prejudicial to safety. Such extreme forms of stress are inherently dangerous, but they have highly beneficial consequences, as well as diet and activity, to stay mild and controlled pressures.

5.2 Enter Polyphenols

So, here's where things get interesting. Many living organisms undergo hormesis, but the reality that this also involves plants is what has been highly undervalued until now. Although we would not typically think of plants as being the same as other living organisms, let alone humans, we do share similar responses in terms of how we respond to our environment on a chemical level.

As mind-blowing as that is, it makes perfect sense to think evolutionary about it, because all living things have adapted to encounter and deal with specific environmental pressures such as starvation, heat, lack of nutrition, and pathogens assault.

If it is hard for you to wrap your head around, get ready for that truly amazing part. Reactions to plant tension are, in general, more complex than ours. Think about it: if we're hungry and thirsty, we can go in search of food and drink; it's too humid, we're in the shade; we can escape under assault. By complete contrast, plants are stagnant, and as such, all the effects of these physiological pressures and challenges will survive. As a consequence, they have built a highly sophisticated stress-response system over the past billion years that humble anything we can boast about. The way they do this is to create a vast collection of natural plant chemicals — called polyphenols— that will help them to adjust to their climate and thrive. We also absorb certain polyphenol nutrients as we eat these products. Their influence is profound: they activate our inherent receptors to react to stress. Here we are talking about precisely the same directions that turn on to fasting and exercise: the sirtuins.

Piggybacking on the stress-response system of a plant in this fashion is regarded as xenohormesis for our gain. And the implications of that are game-changing. Nevertheless, because of their ability to turn on the same positive changes in our bodies, such as fat burning, that would be visible during fasting, these natural plant compounds are now referred to as reflective caloric constraints. And by supplying us with more sophisticated signaling compounds than we are generating ourselves, they cause effects that are comparable to anything that can be obtained by eating or exercising alone.

5.3 Sirt Foods

While all plants have these stress-response systems, only some have evolved to produce remarkable amounts of polyphenols that activate sirtuin. We are naming such plants, Sirtfoods. Their finding suggests there's now a revolutionary new way to trigger the sirtuin genes instead of austere fasting regimens or arduous exercise programs: consuming a rich diet in Sirtfoods. Best of all, this one involves putting Sirtfoods on your dish, not deleting it!

It's so beautifully simple and so quick it seems like a catch is required. But it is not. That is how nature intended us to feed rather than the rumbling stomach or calorie count of the modern diet. Many of you who have endured such hellish diets, where the initial weight reduction is temporary before the body protests, and the weight adds on again, would undoubtedly shudder at the thought of another false promise, another book advertising the infamous "d" term. Yet note this: the current dietary method is just 150 years old; Sirtfoods have been created by evolution about a billion years ago.

And with that, you're still curious to ask what Sirtfoods qualify for specific foods. So here are the top twenty Sirtfoods, without further ado.

SirtFoods	MAJOR SIRTUIN-ACTIVATING NUTRIENTS
Celery with leaves	apigenin
Chilies	luteolin
Parsley	apingenin, myrecitin
Garlic	myrecitin, agoene
Green Tea	epigallocatechin gallate
Kale	kaempferol, quercetin
red endive	luteolin
Red Onion	quercetin
Arugula	quercetin, kaempferol
Cocoa	epicatechin
Extra virgin olive oil	oleuropein, hydroxytyrosol
Walnuts	gallic acid
Buckwheat	rutin
Turmeric	curcumin
Soy	daidzein, formononetin
Strawberries	setin
Capers	kaempferol, quercetin
Dates	gallic acid, caffeic acid
Red wine	resveratrol, piceatannol
Coffee	caffeic acid

SUMMARY

- The belief that fruits, herbs, and plant foods are healthy for us has to be rethought entirely solely because they contain vitamins and antioxidants.

- We are good for us because we contain natural chemicals that put a little stress on our cells, just as fasting and exercise do.

- Plants also built a highly sophisticated stress-response system because they are stationary and created polyphenols to help them respond to their environment's challenges.

- As we consume these products, their polyphenols stimulate our mechanisms of the stress response — our sirtuin genes — emulating the results of caloric restriction and exercise.

- The product with the most sirtuin-activating activity is called Sirtfoods.

Chapter 6: Building a Diet That Works

We were doing something different with the Sirtfood Diet. We took the strongest Sirtfoods on the planet and woven them into a brand-new way of eating, the likes of which were never seen before. We picked the "best of the best" from the healthiest diets we have ever seen and built a world-beating diet from them.

The good news is; you don't immediately have to follow an Okinawan's traditional diet or eat like an Italian mamma. That on the Sirtfood Diet is not only utterly unrealistic but unnecessary. Sure, one thing you might be taken by from the Sirtfoods list is their familiarity. Although you may not consume all of the items on the menu at the moment, you are most definitely eating others. Then why don't you just lose weight already?

The answer is found as we explore the various elements that the most cutting-edge nutrition science indicates are needed to build a workable diet. It is about eating the right amount of Sirtfoods, range, and shape. It's about applying ample protein portions to the Sirtfood plates, and then enjoying your meals at the best time of day. And it's about the right to consume the authentic savory things you love in the amounts you want.

6.1 Hitting Your Quota

Most people just don't eat nearly enough Sirtfoods right now to evoke a strong fat-burning and health-boosting effect. Once researchers looked at the use of five primary nutrient-activating sirtuins (quercetin, myricetin, kaempferol, luteolin, and apigenin) in the US diet, human dietary intakes were found to be miserably 13 milligrams a day. Conversely, the average Japanese consumption was five times greater. Compare this with our Sirtfood Diet experiment, where everyday individuals ate hundreds of milligrams of sirtuin-activating nutrients.

What we are thinking about is a true diet change in which we raise by as much as fifty times our daily intake of sirtuin-activating nutrients. While that may sound overwhelming or unrealistic, it isn't really. Through taking all our top Sirtfoods and bringing them together in a way that is fully compatible with your busy life, you too can quickly and effectively reach the level of consumption required to enjoy all of the benefits.

6.2 Heard a Term 'Synergy'?

We believe it's better to eat a wide range of these wonder nutrients in the form of natural whole grains, where they coexist with the hundreds of other bio-active plant chemicals that act synergistically to improve our wellbeing. We think working for design is more comfortable, rather than against it. It is for this purpose that single nutrient supplements fail to show time and time again.

Take, for example, the classic nutrient resveratrol, which activates sirtuin. In supplement form, it is poorly absorbed; but in its natural food matrix of red wine, its bio availability (how much the body can use) is at least six times higher. Add to this the fact that red wine produces not only one but a whole host of sirtuin activating polyphenols that function together to offer health benefits, including piceatannol, quercetin, myricetin, and epicatechin. Or we could turn our attention from the turmeric to curcumin.

Curcumin is well established to be the critical sirtuin-activating nutrient in turmeric. Yet, research shows that whole turmeric has better PPAR-γ activity for fighting fat loss and is more effective at inhibiting cancer and reducing blood sugar levels than curcumin in isolation. It's not hard to see why isolating a single element in its entire food process is nowhere near as effective as eating it.

But what makes a dietary strategy different is when we start mixing several Sirtfoods. For starters, we are further enhancing the bio availability of resveratrol-containing foods by bringing in quercetin-rich Sirtfoods. Not only this, but they complement each other with their acts. Both are fat busters, but there are variations of how each of them is doing this. Resveratrol is beneficial in helping to kill current fat cells, while quercetin excels in avoiding the formation of new fat cells.6 In addition, all sides target fat, resulting in a more significant impact on the reduction of weight than just eating large amounts of a single food.

And this is a trend which we see again and again. Foods rich in sirtuin activator apigenine improve quercetin absorption from food and enhance its function. Quercetin, in effect, is synergistic with epigallocatechin gallate (EGCG) behavior. Yet EGCG's service with curcumin is synergistic. And so, it begins. Not only are specific whole foods more effective than single ingredients, but we tap into an entire tapestry of health benefits that nature has weaved — so intricate, so pure, it's impossible to try to beat it.

6.3 Juices and Food

Sirtfood Diet is a portion of both juices and whole foods. Here we are thinking about juices explicitly made from a juicer— blenders and smoothie makers (such as the NutriBullet) will not work. For many, this will seem counter intuitive, based on the fact that the fiber is lost when something is juiced. But this is just what we want for leafy greens.

Feed fiber includes what is called non-extractable polyphenols (or NEPPs). These are polyphenols, called sirtuin activators, which are bound to the fibrous portion of the food and only activated by our pleasant gut bacteria until broken down. We don't get the NEPPs by cutting the yarn, so miss out on their beauty. Importantly, though, the NEPP content varies dramatically based on the plant size. The NEPP quality in foods such as meat, cereals, and nuts are substantial and should be consumed whole (NEPPs contain over 50 percent of polyphenols in strawberries!). But for leafy vegetables, the active ingredients in the Sirtfood drink, they are much lower despite having a significant fiber content.

So, when it comes to leafy greens, by juicing them and eliminating the low-nutrient fiber we get full bang for our buck, so we can use even larger volumes and obtain a super concentrated hit of sirtuin-activating polyphenols.

There's another benefit of cutting the thread, too. Leafy greens comprise a form of fiber called insoluble fiber, which has a digestive scrubbing effect. But when we take too much of it, it can irritate and hurt our gut lining just like if we over-scrub stuff. This suggests that for many individuals, leafy green-packed smoothies can overwhelm fiber, possibly aggravating or even inducing IBS (irritable bowel syndrome) and hampering our nutrient absorption.

So, the bottom line is that we need to develop a lifestyle that blends all beverages and whole foods for maximum benefit to get the sirtuin genes going for dramatic weight loss and wellness.

6.4 Power of Protein

It's plants that bring the Sirt into the Sirtfood Diet. However, Sirtfood meals should always be rich in protein to gain maximum benefit. It has been shown that a building block of the dietary protein named leucine has additional benefits in activating SIRT to enhance fat burning and boost blood sugar control.

But leucine also has another part, and this is where it shines through its synergistic partnership with Sirtfoods. Leucine effectively induces anabolism (building things) in our cells, particularly in the muscle, which requires a great deal of energy and ensures that our energy factories (called mitochondria) have to work overtime. It induces a need for the Sirtfoods operation inside our cells. As you may remember, one of the effects of Sirtfoods is to promote the development of more mitochondria, to increase their performance, and to allow them to burn fat as fuel. Our bodies then need these to satisfy this extra demand for energy. The upshot is that we see a synergistic effect when mixing Sirtfoods with dietary protein that enhances sirtuin activation and ultimately gets you to burn fat to support muscle growth and better safety. For this purpose, the meals in the book are built to provide a large protein portion.

Oily fish is an exceptionally good protein alternative to supplement Sirtfoods' action because they are high in omega-3 fatty acids alongside their protein content. There is no way that you will have read a lot about the health benefits of oily fish and especially omega-3 fish oils. And now, recent research suggests that the advantages of omega-3 fats that come from enhancing the functioning of our sirtuin genes.

Over the past few years, many concerns have been raised about the adverse effects of protein-rich diets on wellbeing, and without Sirtfoods to counterbalance the protein, we can start to understand why. Leucine can be a knife with two-edges. We need Sirtfoods, as we have seen, to help our cells fulfill the metabolic demand that leucine imposes upon them. Without them, though, our mitochondria can become unstable, so high levels of leucine will promote obesity and insulin resistance, rather than improve health. Sirtfoods help not only hold the symptoms of leucine in check but also function effectively in our favor.

Speak of leucine as putting the foot on the weight loss and wellness generator, with Sirtfoods, the tool that ensures that the cell satisfies the increased demand. The engine blows, without the Sirtfoods.

Returning to questions about the health effects of protein rich diets, the missing piece of the puzzle is Sirtfoods. Usually, the US diet is protein-rich but requires Sirtfoods to counterbalance it, which makes it essential for Sirtfoods to become an integral part of how Americans live.

6.5 Try to Eat Early

The theory is the sooner, the better when it comes to food, preferably done feeding for the day by 7 p.m. for two significant reasons. Firstly, to harvest the Sirtfoods natural satiating power. Eating a meal that will leave you feeling full, happy, and energized as you go about your day is much more useful than spending the entire day exploring hungry just to feed and remain full while you sleep through the night.

But there's a second good reason to keep eating habits in line with your inner body clock. We also have an internal biological clock, called our circadian rhythm, which controls all of our normal body functions according to day time.

This affects, among other things, how the body handles the food we eat. Our clocks operate in synchrony, above all observing the signals of the sun's light-dark cycle. We're programmed as a diurnal species to be busy in the daytime rather than at night.

The body clock then allows us to handle food more efficiently during the day when it's bright, and we're supposed to be busy, and less so when it's night, where we're primed for rest and sleep instead.

The question is that many of us have "work clocks" and "social clocks," which are not aligned with the sun's slowing down. Sometimes after dark is the only option, some of us get to sleep. To some point, we will teach our body clock in synchronizing with different schedules, including "evening chronotypes" that want or need to be busy, eat and sleep later in the day. Life misaligned from the light-dark environmental process, therefore, comes at a cost.

Research shows that people with evening chronotype have decreased sensitivity to fat gain, muscle loss, and metabolic problems, as well as often suffering from poor sleep. That's just what we see in night shift workers, who have higher rates of obesity and metabolic disease, at least in part due to the impact of their late eating patterns.

The upshot is that when necessary, you're better off eating early in the day, preferably by 7 p.m. but what if that is simply not feasible? The good news is that sirtuins play a crucial part in synchronizing the body clock. Work has found that the polyphenols in Sirtfoods can modulate our body clocks and change circadian rhythm positively. This ensures the addition of Sirtfoods with your meal will mitigate the detrimental effects if you actually cannot avoid eating later on. Yes, one of the frequent comments we receive from Sirtfood Diet adherents is just how much their quality of sleep has increased, indicating the dominant influence on their circadian rhythm harmonization.

6.6 Embrace Eating

Let's give an idea. We just want you to do a very simple thing: don't think about a white bear.

What do you think? For a white bear. Why? For what? As we asked you not to think about it. Don't tell me that you're already there!

This was the trailblazing work conducted by psychology professor Daniel Wegner in 1987 that found that coerced repression of feelings creates a paradoxical and detrimental increase in how often we think about what we are attempting to suppress. So instead of removing it from our minds, the attempt generates a fixation with silenced thinking.

And as you've probably guessed, this trend doesn't just apply to white bears. The same thing happens when we are making heroes and limiting weight loss products.

Studies show that in general, we talk more often about them, rising the urge. It's eating away before we eat it! And now we are much more likely to binge with the diet disrupted and the heightened anxiety about the "forbidden" items we have experienced.

Now the physicists have clarified what's going on here. We all need to be fully autonomous. If we feel restricted, like being on a strict diet, this creates a negative atmosphere, which makes us feel uncomfortable. We get caught up in this misery, and we fight to get free. They protest by doing what we've been advised they shouldn't be doing and doing it a lot more than we would have at first. It happens to us all, even to the most self-controlled people.

It's not a matter of when but if. Researchers also agree that this is a fundamental explanation of why we can sustain diets and even see initial results but struggle to see long-term success.

So, does it really mean that there is no point in even trying to change our eating habits? Are we just doomed to fail? Yes, it implies that we need to create our own optimistic, ideal choice while making a transition to be successful. We already realize that it is not by dietary isolation but through dietary inclusion that we can do it. Instead of concentrating the attention on the disadvantages of what you shouldn't consume, instead, focus on the positive aspects of what you should eat. You avoid the social reaction by doing so. And the Sirtfood Diet's elegance is this. It's about what you bring in your food and not what you're throwing out. It's about consistency and not the amount of your diet.

And it's about you having to do it because you feel satisfied consuming great-tasting foods with the additional awareness that every taste offers a wealth of advantages.

Many diets represent a means to an end. They're about holding in there, trying to keep track of the "healthy dream." However, it rarely comes before the plan stalls, and it's never maintained, even if accomplished. There's a separate Sirtfood Diet. It's all about flying. Phase 1, which reduces calories, is held deliberately short and sweet to ensure positive effects are done before any adverse reaction happens. The emphasis then is entirely on Sirtfoods. And the desire to consume Sirtfoods isn't just motivated by a result of weight loss. But it is just as much if not more about appreciating and loving real food for a safe, active lifestyle.

What's more, once you enjoy Sirtfoods' unique benefits, from fulfilling your hunger to improving your quality of life, you'll see your preferences and tastes change. With the Sirtfood Diet, items that would have previously set off the chain of adverse reactions if you were told that you couldn't consume them would lose their appeal and diminish their influence on you. They become a small part of your diet, and they all met without a single white bear encounter.

SUMMARY

- The Sirtfood Diet draws on the planet's strongest sirtfoods and puts them together practically and straightforwardly to eat.

- It is necessary to eat Sirtfoods in the right amount, mixture, and ways to enjoy the synergistic effects of their sirtuin-activating compounds, in order to achieve optimal results for weight loss and wellbeing.

- Like our modern diets, Sirtfoods stimulates all of our taste receptors, ensuring that we get more satisfaction from our food and feel content sooner.

- By including other healthy ingredients, such as leucine-rich protein foods and oily fish, we further reinforce this to render the results of the Sirtfood Diet even more strong.

- The Sirtfood Diet is an inclusion diet — not isolation, rendering it the only form of diet that can offer weight-loss results over the long term.

Chapter 7: Top-Twenty Sirtfoods

Now that you know everything about Sirtfoods, why they're so powerful, and what it takes to create an effective diet that will deliver lasting results, it's time to get started. The next chapter marks the start of day one of the Sirtfood Diet. So, this is the perfect time to get acquainted with each of the top twenty Sirtfoods, which will soon become the staples of your daily diet.

Arugula

Arugula (also known as rocket, rucola, rugula, and roquette) has a colorful history in American food culture. A pungent green salad leaf with a distinctive peppery taste, it rapidly rose from humble roots to become an emblem of food snobbery in the United States as the source of many peasant dishes in the Mediterranean, thus contributing to the coining of the word arugulance.

But long before it was a salad leaf wielded in a war of class, arugula was known for its medical properties by the ancient Greeks and Romans. Commonly used as a diuretic and digestive aid, it earned its real popularity from its reputation for having strong aphrodisiac powers, so much so that the production of arugula was forbidden in monasteries in the Middle Ages, and the renowned Roman poet Virgil wrote that "the rocket excites the sexual desire of drowsy men." A mixture of kaempferol and quercetin is being studied as a topical product in addition to strong sirtuin-activating effects, as together, they moisturize and promote collagen synthesis in the skin. With those qualifications, it's time to drop the elitist tag and make this the leaf of preference for salad bases, where it beautifully combines with an extra virgin olive oil dressing, combining to create a powerful double act of Sirtfood.

Buckwheat

Buckwheat was one of Japan's earliest domesticated crops, and the story goes that when Buddhist monks made long trips into the mountains, they'd just bring a cooking pot and a buckwheat bag for food. Buckwheat is so nutritious that this was all they needed, and it fed them up for weeks. We're big fans of buckwheat too. Firstly, because it is one of a sirtuin activator's best-known sources, called rutin. But also, because it has advantages as a cover crop, improving soil quality and suppressing weed growth, making it a fantastic crop for environmentally sound and sustainable agriculture.

The explanation buckwheat is head and shoulders above other, more traditional grains is presumably because it's not a grain at all— it's a rhubarb-related fruit crop. Getting one of the highest protein contents of any plant, as well as being a Sirtfood powerhouse, allows it an unrivaled substitute to more widely used grains.

Moreover, it is as versatile as any grain, and being naturally gluten-free, it is a great choice for those intolerant to gluten.

Capers

In case you're not so familiar with capers, we're talking about those salty, dark green, pellet-like things on top of a pizza that you may only have had occasion to see. Yet inevitably, they are one of the most undervalued and overlooked foods out there. Intriguingly, they are the caper bush's flower buds, which grow abundantly in the Mediterranean before being picked and preserved by hand. Studies now reveal that capers possess important antimicrobial, antidiabetic, anti-inflammatory, immunomodulatory, and antiviral properties, and have a history of medicinal use in the Mediterranean and North African regions. It's hardly shocking when we find that they are filled with nutrients that trigger sirtuin.

Celery

For centuries, celery was around and revered — with leaves still adorning the ashes of the Egyptian pharaoh Tutankhamun who died about 1323 BCE. Early strains were very bitter, and celery was generally considered a medicinal plant, especially for cleansing and detoxification to prevent disease. This is especially interesting given that liver, kidney, and gut health are among the many promising benefits that science is now showing. In the seventeenth century, it was domesticated as a vegetable, and selective breeding reduced its strong bitter flavor in favor of sweeter varieties, thus establishing its place as a traditional salad vegetable. It is important to note when it comes to celery, that there are two types: blanched/yellow and Pascal / green. Blanching is a technique developed to reduce the characteristic bitter taste of the celery, which has been perceived to be too strong. This involves shading the celery before harvesting from sunlight, resulting in a paler color and a milder flavor. What a travesty that is, for blanching dumbs down the sirtuin-activating properties of celery as well as dumbing down the taste. Luckily, the tide is changing, and people are demanding true and distinct flavor, turning back to the greener option. Green celery is the sort that we suggest you use in both the green juices and dinners, with the core and leaves being the healthiest pieces.

Chilies

The chili has been an integral part of gastronomic experience worldwide for thousands of years. On one level, it's disconcerting that we'd be so enamored with it. The pungent fire, caused by a substance called capsaicin in chilies, is engineered as a method of plant protection to cause pain and dissuade pests from feasting on it, and we appreciate that. The food and our infatuation with it are almost magical.

Incredibly, one study showed that consuming chilies together even enhances human cooperation.[1] So we know from a health perspective that their seductive fire is wonderful to stimulate our sirtuins so improve our metabolism. The culinary applications of the chili are also endless, making it an easy way to give a hefty Sirtfood boost to any dish.

At times when we appreciate that not everyone is a fan of hot or spicy food, we also hope that we can entice you to consider adding small amounts of chilies, especially in light of recent research showing that those eating spicy foods three or more times a week have a thirteen percent lower death rate compared to those eating them less than once a week.

The hotter the chili, the better its Sirtfood credentials, but be sensitive and stick with what suits your tastes. Serrano peppers are a great start-they tolerable for most people while packing heat. For more experienced heat seekers, we recommend searching for Thai chilies for maximum sirtuin-activating benefits. These can be harder to find in grocery stores but are often found in specialty markets in Asia. Go for deep-colored peppers, excluding those with a wrinkled and fuzzy feel.

Cocoa

Cocoa was considered a holy food and was usually reserved for the elite and the warriors, served at feasts to gain loyalty and duty. Indeed, there was such high regard for the cocoa bean that it was even used as a form of currency. It was normally served as a frothy beverage back then. But what could be a more delicious way to get our dietary quota of cacao than through chocolate?

Unfortunately, there's no count here for the diluted, refined, and highly sweetened milk chocolate we commonly munch. We're talking about chocolate with 85 percent solids of cocoa to earn its Sirtfood badge. But even then, aside from the percentage of cocoa, not every chocolate is created equal. To the acidity to give it a darker color, chocolate is often handled with an alkalizing agent (known as the Dutch process). Sadly, this process diminishes its sirtuin-activating flavanols massively, thereby seriously compromising its health-promoting quality. Fortunately, and unlike in many other countries, food labeling regulations in the United States require alkalized cocoa to be declared as such and labeled "alkali processed." We recommend avoiding these products, even if they boast a higher percentage of cocoa, and opting instead for those who have not undergone Dutch processing to reap the real benefits of cocoa.

Coffee

What's all that about Sirtfood Coffee? We're listening to you. We can assure you that this is no typo. Gone are the days when a twinge of remorse had to balance our love of coffee. The research is unambiguous: coffee is healthy bonafide food. Indeed, it is a real treasure trove of fantastic nutrients that activate sirtuin. And with more than half of Americans drinking coffee every day (to the tune of $40 billion a year!), coffee boasts the accolade of being America's number one source of polyphenols. The ultimate irony is that the one thing we were chastised by so many health "experts" for doing was, in fact, the best thing we were doing for our health each day. This is why coffee drinkers have significantly less diabetes, as well as lower rates of certain cancers and neurodegenerative diseases. As for that ultimate irony, rather than being a toxin, coffee protects our livers and makes them healthier! And on the other hand to the popular belief that coffee dehydrates the body, it is now well established not to be the case, with coffee (and tea) making a perfect contribution to the fluid intake of regular coffee drinkers. So, while we appreciate that coffee is not for everybody, and some people may be susceptible to the effects of caffeine, it's happy days for those who enjoy a cup of joe.

Extra Virgin Olive Oil

Olive oil is the most renowned of Mediterranean traditional diets. The olive tree is among the world's oldest-known planted plants, sometimes established as the "immortal vine." And since people began squeezing olives in stone mortars to collect them, its oil has been revered, almost 7,000 years ago. Hippocrates quoted it as a cure-all; now, a few millennia later, modern science unequivocally asserts its marvelous health benefits. There is now a rich scientific data showing that regular olive oil consumption is highly cardioprotective, as well as playing a role in reducing the risk of major modern-day diseases such as diabetes, certain cancers, and osteoporosis, and associated with increased longevity.

Garlic

Garlic has been considered one of Nature's wonder foods for thousands of years, with healing and rejuvenating powers. Egyptians feed pyramid workers with garlic to enhance their defenses, avoid various diseases, and improve their performance by their ability to prevent exhaustion. Garlic is a natural antibiotic and antifungal that is often used to help treat ulcers in the stomach.

Through facilitating the removal of body waste products, it can activate the lymphatic system to "detox." Besides being investigated for fat loss, it also packs a potent heart health punch, lowering cholesterol by about 10 percent and lowering blood pressure by 5 to 7 percent, as well as lowering blood and blood sugar stickiness. And if you are really concerned about the taste of garlic being off-putting, take note. When women were asked to assess a selection of men's body odors, it was judged that those men who consumed four or more garlic cloves a day had a much more attractive and pleasant smell. Researchers believe this is because it is considered to be a better signal for safety.

And there's always mints for fresher breath, of course!

Green Tea

Many will be acquainted with green tea, the toast of the Orient, and ever more common in the West. As the growing awareness of its health benefits, green tea intake is related to less obesity, heart disease, diabetes, and osteoporosis. The explanation it is believed that green tea is so healthy for us is primarily due to its rich content of a group of powerful plant compounds named catechins, the star of the show is a particular type of sirtuin-activating catechin known as epigallocatechin gallate (EGCG).

What's the fuss about matcha, though? We like to think of matcha on the steroids as normal green tea. In contrast to traditional green tea, which is prepared as an infusion, it is a special powdered green tea which is prepared by dissolving directly in water. The upshot of consuming matcha is that it contains dramatically higher levels of the sirtuin-activating compound EGCG than other green tea types. Zen priests describe matcha as the "ultimate mental and medical remedy that can make one's life more complete" if you are looking for further endorsement.

Kale

We are at heart cynics, so we are always skeptical about what drives the latest craze for superfood advertising. Is it science, or are its interests at stake? In recent years few foods have exploded as dramatically as kale on the health scene. Described as the "lean, green brassica queen" (referring to its cruciferous vegetable family), it has become the chic vegetable for which all health-lovers and foodies are gunning. Each October, there is even a National Day of the Kale. But you don't have to wait until then to show your kale pride: there are also T-shirts, with trendy slogans like "Powered by Kale" and "Highway to Kale." That's enough for us to set the alarm bells ringing.

We've done the research, filled with suspicions, and we have to admit that we conclude that kale deserves her pleasures (although we still don't recommend the T-shirts!). The reason we're pro-kale is that it boasts bumper amounts of the quercetin and kaempferol sirtuin-activating nutrients, making it a must-include in the Sirtfood Diet and the base of our green Sirtfood juice. What's so refreshing about kale is that kale is available everywhere, locally grown, and very affordable, unlike the usual exotic, hard-to-source, and exorbitantly priced so-called superfoods.

Medjool Dates

It may come as a surprise to include Medjool dates in a list of foods that stimulate weight loss and promote health — especially when we tell you that Medjool dates contain a staggering 66 percent sugar. Sugar doesn't have any sirtuin-activating properties at all; rather, it has well-established links to obesity, heart disease, and diabetes — just the opposite of what we're looking to achieve. But processed and replenished sugar is very different from sugar carried in a nature-borne vehicle balanced with sirtuin-activating polyphenols: the date Medjool.

Parsley

Parsley is something of a culinary conundrum. It so often appears in recipes, yet so often it's the green token guy. At best, we serve a couple of chopped sprigs and tossed as an afterthought on a meal, at worst a solitary sprig for decorative purposes only. This way, there on the plate, it is often always languishing even after we have finished eating. This culinary styling stems from its traditional use in ancient Rome as a garnish for eating after meals in order to refresh breath, rather than being part of the meal itself. And what a shame, because parsley is a fantastic food that packs a vibrant, refreshing taste full of character.

Taste aside, what makes parsley special is that it is an excellent source of the sirtuin-activating nutrient apigenin, a real boon since it is seldom found in other foods in significant quantities. In our brains, apigenin binds fascinatingly to the benzodiazepine receptors, helping us to relax and help us to sleep. Stack it all up, and its time we enjoyed parsley not as omnipresent food confetti, but as a food in its own right to reap the wonderful health benefits that it can bring.

Red Endive

Endive is a relatively new kid on the block in so far as vegetables go. The story has it that a Belgian farmer discovered endive in 1830, by accident. The farmer stored chicory roots in his cellar, and then used them as a type of coffee substitute, only to forget them. Upon his return, he discovered that white leaves had sprouted, which he found to be tender, crunchy, and rather delicious upon degustation. Endive is now grown all over the world, including the USA, and earns its Sirtfood badge thanks to its impressive sirtuin activator luteolin content. And besides the established sirtuin-activating benefits, luteolin consumption has become a promising approach to therapy to improve sociability in autistic children.

Note that its texture is crisp and a sweet flavor for those new to endive, accompanied by a gentle and pleasant bitterness. If you're ever stuck on how to increase endive in your diet, you can't lose by adding her leaves to a salad where her welcome, tart flavor adds the perfect bite to an extra virgin olive oil dressing based on zesty. Red is best, just like an onion, but the yellow variety can also be considered a Sirtfood. So while the red type may sometimes be more difficult to find, you should rest assured that yellow is an entirely appropriate substitute.

Red Onions

Since the period of our ancient ancestors, onions have been a dietary staple, being one of the first crops to be grown, around 5,000 years ago. With such a long history of use and such potent health-giving properties, many cultures that came before us have revered onions. They were held especially by the Egyptians as objects of worship, regarding their circle-within-a-circle structure as symbolic of eternal life. And the Greeks assumed that onions make competitors better. Athletes will eat their way through vast amounts of onions before the Olympic Games, also consuming the fruit! It's an incredible testimony to how valuable ancient dietary wisdom can be when we consider that onions earn their top twenty Sirtfood status because they're chock-full of the sirtuin-activating compound quercetin — the very compound that the sports science world has recently started actively researching and marketing to improve sports performance.

And why the red ones? Simply because they have the highest content of quercetin, although the standard yellow ones do not lag too far behind and are also a good inclusion.

Red Wine

Any list of the top twenty Sirtfoods would not be complete without the inclusion of the initial Sirtfood, red wine. The French paradox made headlines in the early 1990s, with it being discovered that despite the French appearing to do everything wrong when it came to health (smoking, lack of exercise, and rich food consumption), they had lower death rates from heart disease than countries like the United States. Physicians proposed the explanation for this was the copious amount of red wine drank. Danish researchers then published work in 1995 to show that low-to-moderate consumption of red wine reduced death rates. In contrast, similar levels of beer alcohol did not affect, and similar intakes of hard liquors increased death rates. Naturally, in 2003, the rich content of red wine from a bevy of sirtuin-activating nutrients was uncovered, and the rest, as they say, was made history.

But there is even more to the impressive resume in red wine. Red wine seems to be able to keep away from the common cold, with moderate wine drinkers having an incidence reduction of more than 40 percent. Research now also shows advantages for oral health and cavity protection. With average consumption, social bonding, and out-of-the-box thinking have also been shown to increase, that after-work drink among colleagues appears to have a basis in solid science to discuss work projects.

Soy

Soy products have a long history as an integral part of the diet of many countries in Asia-Pacific, such as China, Japan, and Korea. Researchers first turned on to soy after finding that high soy-consuming countries had significantly lower rates of certain cancers, particularly breast and prostate cancers. This is thought to be due to a special group of polyphenols in soybeans known as isoflavones, which may favorably change how estrogens work in the body, including daidzein and formononetin sirtuin-activators. Soy product consumption has also been linked to a reduction in the incidence or severity of a variety of conditions such as cardiovascular disease, symptoms of menopause, and bone loss.

Strawberries

In recent years, the fruit has become increasingly vilified, getting a bad rap in the growing fervor toward sugar. Fortunately, such a malignant reputation couldn't be more undeserved for berry-lovers. While all berries are powerhouses of nutrition, strawberries are earning their top twenty Sirtfood status due to their abundance of the fisetin sirtuin-activator. And now, studies support regular eating strawberries to promote healthy growth, keeping off Alzheimer's, obesity, diabetes, heart disease, so osteoporosis. As for their sugar content, a mere teaspoon of sugar per 31/2 ounces is very low.

Intriguingly, and inherently low in sugar itself, strawberries have pronounced effects on how the body handles carbohydrates. What researchers have found is that adding strawberries to carbohydrates reduces the demand for insulin, essentially turning the food into a sustained energy releaser. Yet new research also shows that eating strawberries in diabetes care has similar effects on drug therapy. William Butler, the great physician of the seventeenth century, wrote in praise of the strawberry: "Doubtless God could have made a better berry, but without a doubt, God never did." We can only agree.

Turmeric

Turmeric, a cousin of ginger, is the new kid in food trends on the block, with Google naming it the ingredient of the 2015 breakout star. Although we are only turning to it nowhere in the West, it has been appreciated for thousands of years in Asia, for both culinary and medical reasons. Incredibly, India is producing almost the entire world's turmeric supply, consuming 80 percent of it. In addition to the benefits of the "golden spice" we saw on pages 60–61, in Asia, turmeric is used to treat skin conditions like acne, psoriasis, dermatitis, and rash. Before Indian marriages, there is a ritual where the turmeric paste is added as a skincare treatment to the bride and groom but also to symbolize the warding off darkness.

One factor that prevents turmeric's potency is that its main sirtuin-activating compound, curcumin, is poorly absorbed by the body when we consume it. Research, however, shows that we can overcome this by cooking it in liquid, adding fat, and adding black pepper, all of which increase its absorption dramatically. This fits perfectly with traditional Indian cuisine, wherein curries and other hot dishes it is typically combined with ghee and black pepper, and yet again proves that science only catches up with the age-old wisdom of traditional eating methods.

Walnuts

Dating back to 7000 BCE, walnuts are the oldest known human-made tree food, originating in ancient Persia, where they were the preserve of royalty. Fast forward to the present day, and walnuts are a success story in the US. California is leading the way, with California's Central Valley famous for being the prime walnut-growing area. California walnuts provide the United States with 99 percent of commercial supply and staggering three-quarters worldwide walnut trade.

Walnuts lead the way as the number one nut for safety, according to the NuVal system, which ranks foods according to how nutritious they are and has been endorsed by the American College of Preventive Medicine. But what distinguishes walnuts for us is how they are ay in the face of conventional thinking: they are high in fat and calories, yet well-established to reduce weight and reduce the risk of metabolic diseases such as cardiovascular disease and diabetes. That is the power of activating the sirtuin.

The emerging research showing walnuts to be a powerful anti-aging food is less well known but equally intriguing. Evidence often refers to their advantages as a brain food with the ability to slow down brain ageing and reduce the risk of degenerative brain diseases, as well as reducing the deterioration of physical function with age.

Chapter 8: 7 Pounds in Seven days (Phase 1)

Hello to Sirtfood Diet, Step 1. This is the period of hyper-success, where you will take a massive move in creating a slimmer, leaner body. Follow our easy step-by-step directions and use the delicious recipes you'll find. We also have a meat-free version in addition to our regular seven-day schedule, which is suitable for vegetarians and vegans alike. Feel free to go along with whatever you want.

8.1 What to Expect

You'll enjoy the full benefits of our clinically proven strategy of dropping 7 pounds in seven days during Phase 1. Yet note that involves adding strength, so don't hang up simply with the percentages on the scales. Nor should you become used to measuring yourself every day. In reality, in the last few days of Phase 1, we often see the scales rising due to muscle growth, although waistlines continue to shrink. So, we want you to look at the charts, but not be controlled by them. Find out how you feel inside the mirror, if your clothes fit, or if you need to push a knot on your belt. These are all perfect measures of the underlying shifts in your body composition.

Be mindful of other improvements, too, such as wellbeing, energy levels, and how smooth the skin is. In a local pharmacy, you can even get tests of your general cardiovascular and metabolic wellbeing to see improvements in factors like your blood pressure, blood sugar levels, and blood fats like cholesterol and triglycerides. Also, weight loss aside, incorporating Sirtfoods into your diet is a big step in making your cells fitter and more disease prone, setting you up for an extraordinary balanced lifetime.

8.2 How to Follow Phase 1

We will lead you through the full seven-day program one day at a time to make Phase 1 as plain sailing as possible, including the lowdown on the Sirtfood green juice and easy-to-follow, delicious recipes every step of the way.

This phase of SirtFood Diet has two different stages:

Days 1 to 3 are the most important and you can eat up to a limit of 1000 calories every day during this time, consisting of:

- Three times SirtFood green juices
- One main course

Days 4 to 7 will see the daily intake of food rise to a maximum of 1,500 calories, composed of:

- Two times SirtFood green juices
- Two main courses

There are very few laws with which to obey the diet. Mostly, for lasting progress, it's about incorporating it into the lifestyle and around everyday life. But here are a few easy but big impact tips to get the best result:

1. Take a Good Juicer

Juicing is an essential aspect of the Sirtfood Diet, and a juicer is one of the best health-care purchases you can make. Although price should be the determining factor, certain juicers are more effective at extracting the juice from green leafy vegetables and herbs, with the Breville brand among the best juicers we've tested.

2. Start Preparation

One thing is clear from the multitude of feedback we've had: those who planned ahead of time were the most successful. Get to know the products and techniques, and stock up on what's essential. You'll be amazed at how natural the whole cycle is, with everything planned and ready.

3. Save your Important Time

When time is tight, dress cleverly. Meals can be made the previous night. Juices can be produced in bulk and stored in the refrigerator for up to three days (or longer in the freezer) until their sirtuin-activating nutrient levels begin to fall. Only shield it from light, and only add when you're able to eat it in the match.

4. Eat Early

Eating early in the day is healthier, and hopefully, meals and drinks should not be consumed later than 7 p.m. But the plan is primarily designed to fit the lifestyle, and late eaters always enjoy great benefits.

5. Space Out the Juices

These should be taken at least one hour before or two hours after a meal to maximize the digestion of the green juices and dispersed throughout the day, rather than making them very close together.

6. Eat till You Feel Satisfied

Sirtfood can have dramatic effects on appetite, and some individuals will be satisfied before their meals are over. Hear your body and feed until you're full, instead of forcing down all the calories. Because Okinawans have existed for a long time, it states, "Feed before 80 percent full."

7. Enjoy the Diet

Don't get caught up on the end goal but keep aware of the road instead. This lifestyle is about enjoying food in all its glory, for its health benefits but also for the fun and pleasure it offers. Research shows that we are far more likely to succeed if we maintain our eyes focused on the road rather than the final destination.

8.3 Drinks

As well as the recommended daily portions of green beverages, other drinks can be easy drinking in Phase 1. Non-calorie beverages, usually regular juice, black coffee, and green tea. If your usual tastes are for black or herbal teas, do not hesitate to include these too. Fruit juices and soft drinks are left behind. Alternatively, try adding a few sliced strawberries to still or sparkling water to make your Sirtfood-infused health drink, if you want to spice things up. Hold it for a few hours in the fridge, and you will have a surprisingly cooling option to soft drinks and juices.

One aspect you need to be mindful of is that we don't suggest abrupt, significant changes to your daily coffee use. Caffeine withdrawal symptoms can make you feel bad for a few days; similarly, significant increases may be painful for those especially sensitive to caffeine results. They also recommend drinking coffee without adding milk, because some researchers have found that adding milk will decrease the absorption of the beneficial sirtuin-activating nutrients. The same has been observed with green tea but incorporating any lemon juice increases the absorption of its sirtuin-activating nutrients.

Note that this is the period of hyper-success, and while you should be comforted by the knowledge that it is only for a week, you need to be a little more careful. We have alcohol for this week, in the form of red wine but only as a cooking component.

8.4 The SirtFoods Green Juices

The green juice is an essential part of the Sirtfood Diet's Phase 1 program. All the ingredients are strong Sirtfoods, and in every juice, you get a potent mixture of natural compounds like apigenin, kaempferol, luteolin, quercetin, and EGCG that function together to turn on your sirtuin genes and encourage fat loss. To that, we have attached lemon, as it has been shown that its natural acidity prevents, stabilizes, and improves the absorption of the sirtuin-activating nutrients. We added a touch of apple and ginger to taste too. But both of these are available. Nevertheless, several people find that they take the apple out entirely once they are used to the flavor of the fruit.

SirtFood Green Juices (SERVES 1)

- Two handfuls (about two and a half ounces) kale

- A handful (one ounce or 30g) arugula

- A small handful (about one-fourth ounce or 5g) parsley leaves

- Two to three large celery stalks (five and a half ounces or 150g), including leaves

- Half medium green apple

- Half - to One-inch (1 to 2.5 cm) piece of fresh ginger

- Juice of a half lemon

- Half teaspoon matcha powder*

*Days 1 to 3 of Phase 1: added only to the first two juices of the day

*Days 4 to 7 of Phase 1: added to both juices

Remember that while we weighted all the amounts precisely as described in our pilot experiment, our experience is that a handful of measures work exceptionally well. In reality, they are the best tailoring the number of nutrients to the body size of a person. More significant people tend to have more massive paws, and thus get a proportionally higher volume of Sirtfood nutrients to suit their body size and vice versa for smaller people.

- Bring together the greens (kale, arugula, and parsley), and blend them. We consider juicers may vary in their efficacy when juicing leafy vegetables, and you may need to rejuice the remains before going on to the other ingredients. The goal is to end up with around 2 ounces of material, or about 1/4 cup (50ml) of green juice.

- Now, blend the Celery, apple, and ginger.

- You should cut the lemon and also bring it through the juicer, but we find it much easier to push the lemon into the juice by hand. You should have about 1 cup (250ml) of juice in total by this point, perhaps somewhat more.

• It's only when you extract the juice and are ready to serve that you add the matcha. In a bowl, pour a tiny amount of juice, then add the matcha, and mix vigorously with a fork or whisk. In the first two beverages of the day, we only use matcha, because it includes small amounts of caffeine (the same quality as a regular teacup). When wasted late, it can keep you awake with those not used to it.

• After the matcha is resolved, add the juice that left. Give it a final blend, and the juice is ready to drink. Easy to top up with plain water, as you like.

For Days 1 – 3, you can take the juices at different times of the day, and then you can take on a standard meal, eat it at a time that suits you (preferably eaten for lunch or dinner).

DAY 1

• Three times Sirtfood green juices

• One main course either;

Fried shrimps with Buckwheat noodles + one-fourth chocolate bar

Or

Miso and sesame glazed tofu with ginger and chili stir-fried greens + one-fourth chocolate bar

DAY 2

• Three times Sirtfood green juices

• One main course either;

Turkey with capers and parsley and spiced cauliflower + one-fourth chocolate bar

Or

Kale and red onion with buckwheat (vegan) + one-fourth chocolate bar

DAY 3

- Three times Sirtfood green juices

- One main course either;

Chicken breast piece with kale, red onion, and red salsa + one-fourth chocolate bar

Or

Harissa baked tofu with spiced cauliflower + one-fourth chocolate bar

> For Days 4-7, you can take the juices at different times of the day, and then you can take on a standard meal, eat it at a time that suits you (preferably eaten for breakfast/lunch or dinner). But as per your appetite, you can continue to add in half to three-fourth ounce (15g to 20g) dark chocolate, each day at your discretion.

DAY 4

- Two times Sirtfood green juices

- Two main courses either;

MEAL ONE: Sirt Muesli

MEAL TWO: Pan-fried Salmon fillet with caramelized endive, arugula and Celery leaves salad

Or

MEAL ONE: Sirt Muesli (vegan)

MEAL TWO: Tuscan bean stew (vegan)

DAY 5

- Two times Sirtfood green juices

- Two main courses either;

MEAL ONE: Strawberry buckwheat (vegan)

MEAL TWO: Buckwheat noodles in a miso broth with tofu, Celery, and kale (vegan)

Or

MEAL ONE: Strawberry buckwheat (vegan)

MEAL TWO: Marinated miso with stir-fried greens and sesame

DAY 6

- Two times Sirtfood green juices

- Two main courses either ;

MEAL ONE: Sirt super salad

MEAL TWO: Grilled beef with red wine, onion rings, garlic kale, and herb-roasted potatoes

Or

MEAL ONE: Lentil sirt super salad (vegan)

MEAL TWO: Bean mole with bakes potatoes (vegan)

DAY 7

- Two times Sirtfood green juices

- Two main courses either;

MEAL ONE: Sirtfood omelet

MEAL TWO: Chicken breast (baked) with parsley pesto and red onion salad

Or

MEAL ONE: Sirt super salad (vegan)

MEAL TWO: Roasted eggplant wedges with walnut and parsley pesto and red onion salad (vegan)

Chapter 9: Maintenance

Congratulations on completing Sirtfood Diet Step 1! You should already have excellent results of fat loss and not only appear slimmer and more toned but also feel revitalized and re-energized. Okay, now what?

Having seen these sometimes-incredible changes ourselves, we realize how much you're going to want to see much better results, not just retain all those advantages. Sirtfoods are, after all, designed to eat for life. The problem is how you adapt what you learned in Phase 1 into your regular dietary practice. That is precisely what inspired us to develop a fourteen-day maintenance plan designed to help you make the transition from Phase 1 to your more usual dietary regimen, thus helping to maintain and expand the benefits of the Sirtfood Diet further.

9.1 What to Expect

You should maintain the weight loss results through Phase 2 and continue to lose weight gradually. Also, the one striking thing we've seen with the Sirtfood Diet is that most or all of the weight people lose is from fat and that many put some muscle on. So, we would like to warn you again not to measure your success solely based on the numbers. Look in the mirror to see if you look leaner and more toned, see how well your clothes fit and lap up the compliments you'll get from others.

Note that just as weight loss occurs, the health benefits will increase. In implementing the fourteen-day maintenance plan, you are helping to lay the foundations for a lifelong health future.

9.2 How to Follow Phase 2

The key to success in this process is having your diet packed full of Sirtfoods. We've put together a seven-day meal schedule for you to adapt to make it as easy as possible, with tasty family-friendly meals, filled with Sirtfoods every day to the rafters. Now what you need to do is to implement Seven Day Program twice to fulfill Phase 2's fourteen days.

On each of fourteen days, your diet will consist of:

- Three times balanced sirtfood meals
- 1-time sirtfood green juice
- 1 – 2 times optional sirtfood snacks

Also, when you have to eat those, there are no strict laws. Be agile throughout every day and suit them. Two basic thumb-rules are:

- Take sirtfood green juice either in the morning or at least half an hour before breakfast.
- Try your best to take dinner by 7 PM.

9.3 Portion Sizes

In Phase 2, our attention is not on calorie counting. For the average person, this is not a practical approach or even a good one over the long term. Instead, we concentrate on healthy servings, really well-balanced meals, and most notably, filling up on Sirtfoods so that you can continue to benefit from their fat-burning and health-promoting impact.

We've even designed the meals in the plan to make them satiate, making you stay full for longer. This coupled with Sirtfoods' innate appetite-regulating power, ensures you're not going to spend the next 14 days feeling thirsty, but rather comfortably fulfilled, well-fed, and highly well-nourished.

Just like in Phase 1, try to listen and be driven by your appetite. When you prepare meals according to our guidelines and notice that you are easily full before you finish a meal, then stop eating is perfectly fine!

9.4 What to Drink

During Phase 2 you'll need to include one green juice every day. This is to keep you top with high Sirtfoods prices.

Just like in Phase 1, you will easily absorb other fluids in Phase 2. Our preferred beverages contain remaining plain water, bottled flavored water, coffee, and green tea. Whether black or white tea is your preference, feel free to enjoy it. The same goes for herbal teas. The best news is that during Phase 2, you will enjoy the occasional bottle of red wine. Due to its content of sirtuin-activating polyphenols, particularly resveratrol and piceatannol, red wine is a sirtfood that makes it the best choice of alcoholic beverage. However, with alcohol itself causing adverse effects on our fat cells, restraint is still safest, so we suggest restricting the drink to one glass of red wine with a meal for two to three days a week in Phase 2.

9.5 Returning to Three Meals

You enjoyed only one or two meals per day during Phase 1 and allowed you plenty of versatility when you eat your meals. As we are now back to a more normal routine and the well-tested practice of three meals a day, learning about breakfast is a good time.

Eating a good breakfast sets, us on for the day, raising our levels of energy and focus. Eating early holds our blood sugar and fat rates in balance, in terms of our metabolism. The breakfast is a good thing that is pointed out by a number of studies, usually showing that people who eat breakfast often are less prone to overweight.

The explanation for this is because of our internal clocks inside. Our bodies are asking us to feed early in expectation of when we will be most busy and need food. Yet, as many as a third of us will miss breakfasts on any given day. It's a classic symptom in our crazy modern life, and the feeling is there's simply not enough time to eat properly. But as you will see, with the nifty breakfasts we have laid out for you here, nothing could be further from the truth. Whether it's the Sirtfood smoothie that can be drunk on the go, the premade Sirt muesli, or the quick and easy Sirtfood scrambled eggs/tofu, finding those extra few minutes in the morning will reap dividends not only for your day but for your longer-term weight and health.

With Sirtfoods functioning to overcharge our energy levels, there's, even more, to learn from getting a hit from them early in the morning to continue your day. This is done not only by consuming a Sirtfood-rich meal but above all by including the green juice, which we suggest you have either first thing in the morning — at least thirty minutes before breakfast— or mid-morning. We get a lot of reports from our personal experience of people who first consume their green juice and don't feel hungry for a few hours afterward. If this is the impact it's having on you, taking a couple of hours until having breakfast is perfectly fine. Just don't miss this one. Instead, with a good breakfast, you should kick off your day, then wait two to three hours to have the green juice. Be versatile, and just go with anything that suits you.

9.6 Sirtfood Snacks

You should keep it when it comes to snacking or quit it. There is a long debate on about whether consuming regular, smaller meals is better for weight loss, or just keeping to three balanced meals a day. The fact is, that does not matter.

The way we've designed the maintenance menu for you means you're going to eat three well-balanced Sirtfood-rich meals a day, and you may notice that you don't need a snack. But maybe you've been busy with the kids in the classroom, working out or dashing about and need something to take you into the next meal. And if that "little something" is going to give you a whammy of Sirtfood nutrients and taste delicious, then it's happy days. This is why we created our "Sirtfood bites." These smart little snacks are a genuinely guilt-free treat made entirely from Sirtfoods: dates, walnuts, cocoa, extra virgin olive oil, and turmeric. We recommend eating one, or a maximum of two, per day for the days when you require them.

9.7 Sirtifying Your Meal

We saw that the only consistent diets are those of participation, not exclusion. Yet real success goes beyond this— the diet has to be consistent with living in modern days. Whether it's the ease of meeting the demands of our hectic lives or fitting in with our position at dinner parties as to the bon vivant, the way we eat should be trouble-free. You will appreciate your svelte body and beautiful smile, rather than thinking about the demands and limitations of kooky products.

What makes Sirtfoods so great is that they are available, common, and simple to include in your diet. Below, when you bridge the gap between step 1 and daily feeding, you can lay the foundations for a modern, better lifelong eating strategy.

The key principle is what we term the meals "Sirtifying." This is where we take popular meals, including many traditional classics, and we retain all the great taste with some smart modifications and easy Sirtfood inclusions but attach a lot of goodness to that. You'll see just how quickly this is done in Phase 2.

Highlights include our tasty smoothie Sirtfood for the ultimate on-the-go breakfast in a time-consuming environment and the easy turn from wheat to buckwheat to add extra flavor and zip to the much-loved pasta comfort food. While classic, famous dishes such as chili con carne and curry don't even need much improvement, with Sirtfood bonanzas providing traditional recipes. Yet who has said that fast food means bad health? If you prepare something yourself, we mix the true vivid tastes of a pizza and through the shame. There's no need to say goodbye to indulgence yet, as our smothered pancakes with berries and dark chocolate sauce have demonstrated. It's not even a treat, it's breakfast, and for you it's perfect. Simple changes: you keep eating the things that you enjoy when maintaining healthy weight and well-being. And that is Sirtfoods, the culinary movement.

9.8 Fourteen-Day Meal Plan

Beyond our standard plan, we also have a meat-free version which is suitable for vegetarians as well as vegans. You can also mix it with whatever you want.

Each day you will consume

- Three times balanced sirtfood meals
- 1-time sirtfood green juice
- 1 – 2 times optional sirtfood snacks

BREAKFAST

Days	Breakfast
Day 1 & Day 8	Sirtfood Smoothie
Day 2 & Day 9	Sirt Muesli
Day 3 & Day 10	Yogurt with mixed walnuts, and dark choc OR coconut yogurt with chopped walnuts, and d
Day 4 & Day 11	Spiced scrambled egg
Day 5 & Day 12	Sirtfood smoothie
Day 6 & Day 13	: Buckwheat pancakes chocolate sauce, and cr OR coconut yogurt with chopped walnuts, and d
Day 7 & Day 14	Sirtfood Omelet or Sirt

LUNCH & DINNER

Lunch	Dinner
1. Chicken Sirt super salad	Asian shrimp stir-f noodles
2. Waldorf salad	Tuscan bean stew
3. Stuffed whole-wheat pita	Butternut squash an buckwheat
4. Butter bean and miso dip with celery sticks and oatcakes	Butternut squash an buckwheat
5. Tuna Sirt super salad	Chicken and kale potatoes
6. Stuffed whole-wheat pita	Kale and red onion dal
7. Strawberry buckwheat tabbouleh	Sirt chili con carne
8. Strawberry buckwheat tabbouleh	Kidney bean mole with

9. Waldorf salad	Smoked salmon pasta ˅
10. Buckwheat pasta salad	Harissa baked tofu witl
11. Tofu and shiitake mushroom soup	Sirtfood pizza
12. Tofu and shiitake	Mushroom soup
13. Lentil Sirt super salad	Baked chicken breas parsley pesto and red c
14. Lentil Sirt super salad	Miso and sesame glaze chill stir-fried greens

Chapter 10: Sirtfoods for Life

Congratulations, all stages of the Sirtfood Diet have now finished! Just let's take stock of what you have achieved. You've entered the hyper-success process, achieving weight loss in the area of 7 pounds, which probably includes an attractive increase in muscle. You also maintained your weight loss throughout the fourteen-day maintenance phase and further strengthened the body composition. Perhaps notably, you have marked the beginning of your transformation of wellness. You took a stand against the tide of ill health, which strikes so often as we get older. The life you have decided for yourself is enhanced strength, productivity, and health.

By now, you'll be familiar with the top twenty Sirtfoods, and you've gained a sense of how powerful they are. Not only that, you'll probably have become quite good at including them in your diet and loving them. For the sustained weight loss and health, they offer, these items must stay a prominent feature in your everyday eating regimen. But still, they're just twenty foods, and after all, the spice of life is variety. What next, then? We'll give you the blueprint for lifelong health in this chapter.

It's about getting your body in perfect balance with a diet that's suitable and sustainable for everyone and providing all the nutrients we need that enhance our health. It's about keeping on reaping the Sirtfood Diet's weight-loss rewards using the very best foods nature has to offer.

10.1 Some other Sirtfoods

We've seen why Sirtfoods are so beneficial: certain plants have sophisticated stress-response mechanisms that generate compounds that trigger sirtuins— the same fasting and exercise-activated fat-burning and durability mechanism in the body. The greater the quantity of these compounds generated by plants in response to stress, the greater the value we derive from their feeding. Our list of the top twenty Sirtfoods is made up of the foods that stand out because they are particularly packed full of these compounds, and hence the foods that have the most exceptional ability to impact body composition and wellbeing. But foods ' sirtuin-activating results aren't a concept of all or nothing. There are many other plants out there that produce moderate levels of sirtuin-activating nutrients, and by eating these liberally, we encourage you to expand the variety and diversity of your diet. The Sirtfood Diet is all about inclusion, and the greater the range of sirtuin-activating items that can be integrated into the diet. Especially if that means you will obtain from your meals even more of your favorite foods to increase pleasure and enjoyment.

Let's use the workout comparison. The top twenty Sirtfoods are the (much more pleasurable) equivalent of sweating it out at the gym, with Phase 1 being the "boot camp." By contrast, eating those other foods with more moderate levels of sirtuin-activating nutrients is like reaping the rewards of going out for a good walk. Contrast that to the typical diet that has a nutritional value equal to sitting all day on the couch watching Television. Yeah, sweating it out in the gym is fine, but if that is all you do, you will quickly get fed up with it. The walk should also be welcomed, especially if it means that you don't just choose to sit on the sofa.

For e.g., in our top twenty Sirtfoods, we have included strawberries because they are the most prominent source of the sirtuin activator fisetin. Yet if we look more broadly at berries as a food group, we find that they have metabolic health benefits as well as healthy ageing. Reviewing their nutritional content, we note that other berries such as blackberries, black currants, blueberries, and raspberries also have significant amounts of nutrients that cause sirtuins.

The same holds with nuts. Notwithstanding their calorific material, nuts are so effective that they promote weight loss and help shift inches from the waist. This is in addition to cutting chronic disease risk. Though walnuts are our champion nut, nutrients that trigger sirtuin can also be found in chestnuts, pecans, pistachios, and even peanuts.

Instead, we turn our attention to food. Throughout recent years there has been in several areas an increasing aversion to grains. Studies, however, link whole grain consumption with decreased inflammation, diabetes, heart disease, and cancer. Although they do not equal the pseudo-grain buckwheat Sirtfood qualifications, we do see the existence of substantial sirtuin-activating nutrients in other whole grains. And needless to say, their sirtuin-activating nutrient quality is decimated when whole grains are converted into refined "clean" forms. Such modified models are quite dangerous groups and are interested in a number of state-of-the-art health problems. We're not saying you can never eat them, but instead, you're going to be much better off sticking to the whole-grain version whenever possible.

With the likes of goji berries and chia seeds possessing Sirtfood powers, also notorious "superfoods" get on the bandwagon. That is most likely the unwitting reason for the health benefits they have observed. While it does imply that they are healthy for us to consume, we do know that there are easier, more available, and better options out there, so don't feel compelled to get on that specific bandwagon! We see the same trend across a lot of food categories. Unsurprisingly, the foods that research has developed are usually good for us, and we should be consuming more of them. Below we mentioned about forty foods that we discovered have Sirtfood properties too. We actively encourage you to include these foods to maintain and continue your weight loss and wellbeing as you expand your diet repertoire.

Vegetables

- artichokes
- asparagus
- broccoli
- frisée
- green beans
- shallots
- watercress
- white onions
- yellow endive

Fruits

- apples
- blackberries
- black currants
- black plums
- cranberries
- goji berries
- kumquats
- raspberries
- red grapes

Nuts and seeds

- chestnuts
- chia seeds
- peanuts
- pecan nuts
- pistachio nuts
- sunflower seeds

Grains and pseudo-grains

- popcorn
- quinoa

• whole-wheat flour
Beans

• fava beans
• white beans (e.g., cannellini or navy)
Herbs and spices

• chives
• cinnamon
• dill (fresh and dried)
• dried oregano
• dried sage
• ginger
• peppermint (fresh and dried)
• thyme (fresh and dried)

Beverages
• black tea
• white tea

10.2 Power of Protein

A high protein diet is one of the most popular diets of the last few years. Higher protein intake while dieting has been shown to encourage satiety, sustain metabolism, and reduce muscle mass loss. But it's when they pair Sirtfoods with protein that things get brought to a whole new level. Protein is, as you may remember, a necessary addition in a diet based on Sirtfood to gain maximum benefits. Protein consists of amino acids, and it is a particular amino acid, leucine, which effectively complements Sirtfoods ' behavior, strengthening their effects. This is done primarily by changing our cellular environment so that our diet's sirtuin-activating nutrients work much more effectively. It ensures we get the best result from a Sirtfood-rich meal, which is paired with protein-based in leucine. Leucine's main dietary sources contain red meat, pork, fruit, vegetables, milk, and dairy products.

10.3 Animal Based-Protein

Animal products have been implicated in recent years as a contributing cause of many Western diseases, especially cancer. If that is the case, eating them with Sirtfoods may not sound like such a bright idea. Here's our lowdown to lay that to rest.

One of the significant concerns regarding milk is that it is not just a simple food but a highly sophisticated signaling mechanism to cause rapid offspring body production. Although this has a cherished meaning in early life, it may not be so common in adult life. Persistent and hyper activating the primary growth signal now correlated with ageing and the progression of age-related disorders such as obesity, type 2 diabetes, cancer, and neurodegenerative diseases. Notwithstanding the intricacies of this signaling system being a relatively new area of research and thus still very much an uncertain and theoretical possibility, this does explain why people might shy away from dairy products. However, the study points to one thing: if we add Sirtfoods to a dairy-containing diet, they inhibit mTOR's inappropriate effects on our cells, rescind this risk, making Sirtfoods a must-include with a dairy-based diet.

Generally, there are mixed reviews of the association between dairy and cancer. If we stack up all the study, mild dairy consumption is perfectly fine in the sense of a Sirtfood-rich diet and can deliver several useful nutrients to supplement Sirtfoods.

Poultry is ok when it comes to meat and cancer risk, but red and fried meats are much more suspect. Although data concerning them in breast and prostate cancer on the field is pretty thin, there is a legitimate concern that red and processed meat eating plays a role in intestinal cancer. Processed meat, such as sausages tends to be the worst perpetrator. Although there is no need to take it off the table, it should be included in just small amounts, rather than being a constant.

The good news for red meat is that research shows that cooking it with Sirtfoods rescues the risk of cancer, whether it's making a marinade with herbs, seasoning, and extra virgin olive oil; frying the beef with onions, or simply adding a nice cup of green tea to the meal or indulging in dark chocolate after dinner.

These all pack a punch from Sirtfood, which helps to neutralize the harmful effects of red meat. While we're all out to have the steak and consume it, don't go crazy. Red meat consumption is best kept at around 1 pound (500 g) per week (cooked weight), roughly equivalent to 1.5 pounds (700 to 750 g) fresh.

The link between egg consumption and cancer risk has not been investigated as extensively as meat and dairy products have, but there seems little cause for concern in this regard. Which eggs have been active in inducing is heart disease, instead? This is because they constitute a significant dietary cholesterol source. Thus, we are advised to restrict the use of eggs. Further countries, including Nepal, benefit interestingly. Who is right, then? The reason for siding with the latter is compelling. There is no linked routine egg intake with any increased risk of coronary heart disease or stroke. Although specific genetic disorders that involve a decreased consumption of dietary cholesterol, this limitation is not appropriate for the general population.

10.4 The Power of Three

The omega-3 long-chain fatty acids EPA and DHA are the second major category of nutrients that effectively complement Sirtfoods. Omega-3s have been the coveted natural wellbeing global favorite for years. What we didn't know before, which we are doing now, is that they also improve the activation of a group of sirtuin genes in the body that is directly linked to longevity. It makes them the perfect match for Sirtfoods.

Omega-3s have potent effects in decreasing inflammation and lowering fat blood levels. To that, we can add additional heart-healthy effects: rendering the blood less likely to pool, stabilizing the heart's electrical activity, and lowering blood pressure. Even the pharmaceutical industry now looks to them as an aid in the war against cardiac disease. And that is not where the litany of benefits ends. Omega-3s also have an effect on the way we perceive, having been shown to boost the outlook and help stave off dementia.

When we speak about omega-3s, we're thinking primarily about eating fish, particularly oily types, because no other dietary source comes close to supplying the significant levels of EPA and DHA that we need. And to see the benefits, all we need is two servings of fish a week, with an emphasis on oily fish. Sadly, the United States is not a country of big fish eaters, and that is accomplished by less than one in five Americans. As a result, our intake of the precious EPA and DHA is appallingly short.

Plant foods, including almonds, beans, and green leafy vegetables, often produce omega-3 but in a form called alpha-linolenic acid, which must be processed into EPA or DHA in the body. This conversion process is poor, meaning that alpha-linolenic acid delivers a negligible amount of our needs for omega-3. Even with the wonderful advantages of Sirtfoods, we shouldn't forget the added value that drinking adequate omega-3 fats provides. In that order, the best sources of omega-3 fish are herring, sardines, salmon, trout, and mackerel. While fresh tuna is naturally high, too, the tinned version loses the majority of the omega-3. And a replacement of DHA-enriched microalgae (up to 300 milligrams a day) is also recommended for vegetarians and vegans, though food foods should still be integrated into the diet.

10.5 Can A SirtFood Provide it All?

Our focus so far has been solely on Sirtfoods and reaping their maximum benefits in order to achieve the body we want and powerfully boost our health in the process. But is this a reasonable, long-term dietary solution to be taken? After all, there is more to diet than pure nutrients that trigger sirtuin. What about all the vitamins, minerals, and fibers that are also important to our wellbeing, and the diets that we should consume to satisfy such demands?

Based on sirtfood diets, augmented by protein-rich foods and omega-3 outlets, fulfill dietary needs across the entire spectrum of essential nutrients— much more so than any other diet does. They use kale, for example, because it is a good sirtfood, but it is a great source of vitamins C, folate, and manganese, calcium, Vitamin K and magnesium minerals. Kale is also a tremendous source of carotenoids lutein and zeaxanthin, both of which are critical for eye health, as well as immune-boosting beta-carotene.

Walnuts are also rich in minerals such as magnesium, copper, zinc, manganese, calcium, and iron, as well as fiber. Buckwheat is made of manganese, magnesium, zinc, potassium, and cotton. Tick the boxes of the onions for vitamin B6, folate, potassium, and food. Yet bananas, as well as potassium yet manganese, are good sources of vitamin C. And so, it begins. When you broaden your menu to include the expanded Sirtfood list and leave space for all the other good foods you enjoy eating, unwittingly, what you're going to end up with is a diet that's far richer in vitamins, nutrients, and fiber than you've ever had before. What Sirtfoods offers is a missing food group that changes the landscape of how we judge how good foods are for us, and how we eat a genuinely full diet.

10.6 The Physical Activity Effect

The Sirtfood Diet is about consuming certain products that are designed to promote sustainable weight loss and wellbeing by definition. But with the advantages that you see by practicing the plan, you can fall into the trap of feeling there's no need to exercise. This will be endorsed by many diet books, saying how ineffective exercise is compared with following the right diet for weight loss. And it's real; we can't outdo a bad diet. It's not the approach we saw earlier that was supposed to support weight loss. It's inefficient, and the harmfulness of being too many borders. So, it's that till we see stars or achieve an Olympian's feats, there's no need to pound the treadmill — but what about general everyday movement?

The truth is we are now much less involved than we used to be. The age of technology has ensured physical activity is practically factored out of our daily lives, for all the advancements it has provided. We don't have to mess with the whole process of being involved unless we want to. We can roll out of bed, drive to work, take the elevator, sit at a desk the whole day, drive home, eat and watch TV before rolling back into bed, then do the same the next day and the next day.

Forget about weight loss for a second and just glance at the litany of positive health benefits correlated with it. These include reduced risk of cardiovascular disease, stroke, hypertension, type 2 diabetes, osteoporosis, obesity and cancer, and improved mood, sleep, confidence, and a sense of wellbeing.

While many of the benefits of being active are driven by switching on our sirtuin genes, eating Sirtfoods shouldn't be used as a reason to not engage in exercise. Instead, we should understand how active the ideal complement to our Sirtfood intake is. It activates optimum stimulation of the sirtuin, and all the advantages that it provides, just as expected by definition.

What we are talking about here is meeting 150-minute (2 hours and 30 minutes) government guidelines of moderate physical activity a week. A moderate job is the equivalent of a brisk walk. But that doesn't have to be limited to this. Any sport or physical activity you love is fitting. Pleasure and exercise do not have to be mutually exclusive! So, their social aspect enriches squad or group sports even more. It's also about everyday things like taking the bike instead of the car, or getting off the bus one stop earlier, or just parking farther away to increase the distance you've got to walk around. Take the stairs and not the lift. Go outdoors and do gardening. Play in the park with your kids or get more out with the dog. Everything counts. Everything that has you up and moving will activate your sirtuin genes regularly and at moderate intensity, enhancing the benefits of the Sirtfood Diet.

Engaging in physical activity and eating a diet high in Sirtfood brings the buck the full sirtuin click. All it takes to achieve the benefit of physical activity is the equivalent of a quick 30-minute stroll five days a week.

SUMMARY

- Although the top twenty Sirtfoods should remain at the center of the plate, there are many other plants with sirtuin-activating properties that should be included in our diets to make them diverse and varied.

- A diet rich in Sirtfoods augmented by the addition of animal products and seafood offers all the advantages of triggering sirtuin, as well as satisfying the need for other essential nutrients.

- Although vegans and vegetarians can get all the benefits from a diet based on Sirtfood, careful attention should be paid to those nutrients that may be deficient, and correct food choices or supplements should be created.

Questions & Answers

1.   If I am not fat, can I still follow this diet?

For anyone who is underweight, we do not prescribe Step 1 of the Sirtfood Diet. A simple way to find out that if you are underweight is to measure the body mass index. As long as you are aware of your height and weight, you can quickly determine using any number of online BMI calculators. If your BMI is 18 or less, we do not recommend embarking on the diet phase 1. They would still urge caution if your BMI is between 18.5 and 20, as adopting the diet can imply that your BMI drop below 18.5. While many people aspire to be super-skinny, the reality is that underweight can have a negative impact on many health aspects, contributing to a lower immune system, an increased risk of osteoporosis (weakening bones), and fertility issues. While phase 1 of the diet is not recommended if you are underweight, we still encourage the integration of plenty of Sirtfoods into a balanced way of eating so that all the health benefits of these foods can be reaped. If you're slim but have a healthy range of BMI (20–25), however, there's absolutely nothing to stop you from getting started. A majority of the pilot trial participants had BMI in the healthy range, but still lost impressive amounts of weight and got more toned. Importantly, many of them reported significantly improved levels and appearance of the energy. Sirtfood diet is about promoting health just as much as weight-loss.

2.   If you take any medications, so is it fine to follow this diet?

The Sirtfood Diet is suitable for most people. Still, due to its powerful effects on fat burning and health, it can alter the processes of certain diseases and the medication actions prescribed by your doctor. Similarly, certain medicines are not suitable in a state of fasting. During the Sirtfood Diet trial, we assessed each individual's suitability before they embarked on the diet, particularly those taking medication. We can't do that for you, so if you have a significant health problem, are taking prescribed medicines or have other reasons to worry about getting on a diet, we recommend that you discuss it with your doctor.

3.   If someone's expecting, still can follow this diet?

If you are trying to conceive or are pregnant or breastfeeding, we do not recommend embarking on the Sirtfood Diet. It is a powerful diet for weight loss which makes it inappropriate. Don't be put off eating plenty of Sirtfoods, though, as these are exceptionally healthy foods to be included as part of a balanced and varied pregnancy diet. Because of its alcohol content, you will want to avoid red wine and limit caffeinated items such as coffee, green tea, and cocoa not to exceed 200 milligrams of caffeine per day during pregnancy (one mug of instant coffee typically contains about 100 milligrams of caffeine). Recommendations should not surpass four cups of green tea per day and should skip matcha altogether. Other than that, you can reap the benefits of incorporating sirt foods into your diet.

4.   How often can I repeat Phase 1 and Phase 2?

Phase 1 can be repeated if you feel a weight loss or health boost is needed. To ensure long-term adverse effects of calorie restriction on your metabolism are not present, you should wait at least a month before repeating. But in fact, we find that most people at most need to repeat in no more frequently than once in every three months and continue to get incredible results. Instead, if you find that you've gone off-track, need some fine-tuning, or want a bit more sirtfood intensity, we recommend repeating as often as you like some or all days of the Phase 2 section. Phase 2 is, after all, about establishing a lifelong way to eat. Remember, the Sirtfood Diet's beauty is that it doesn't require you to feel like you're endlessly on a diet. Still, instead, it's the springboard to developing positive lifelong dietary changes that create a lighter, leaner, healthier you.

5. I have heard many times about superfoods, should I include these in my diet?

The first thing you need to know about the term superfood is that it's a marketing slogan and not a scientific term at all. You don't need to think about so-called superfoods because the Sirtfood Diet puts together the planet's healthiest foods into a revolutionary new way of eating. Just as relying on a simple vitamin pill to make us healthy is a mistake, so building on a single superfood to do the same is also a mistake. It is the entire diet, consisting of a broad spectrum of Sirtfoods and their vast array of natural compounds, acting in synergy, which is the real secret to achieving weight loss and lifelong health.

6. Should I exercise during Phase 1?

Regular exercising is the best things you can do for your health and doing some moderate exercise will enhance the diet's phase 1 weight-loss and health benefits. In general, we advise you to maintain your usual level of exercise and physical activity through the Sirtfood Diet's first seven days. However, we suggest staying in your normal comfort zone, as prolonged or excessively intense exercise can simply put too much stress on the body during this period. Eye your body. There's no need to push yourself during Phase 1 for more exercise; instead, let the Sirtfoods do the hard work.

7. I am fat, is sirtfood diet best for me?

Yeah! Don't be upset by the fact that only a small minority of our pilot study participants were obese. This is because the pilot study was conducted in a health and fitness club where people are usually fitter and more aware of their well-being. Instead, be encouraged by the fact that the few who were obese had even better results than our healthy-weight participants. There are a lot of people of people who tried the diet in the real world replicated those results. You should also stand to reap the most significant changes in your well-being, based on the research into sirtuin activation. Getting obese increases the risk of many chronic health problems, and these are the very diseases against which Sirtfoods helps to protect.

8.   If I get the best results and reached my target weight, so should I stop eating sirtfoods?

Firstly, many congratulations on your success in terms of weight loss! With Sirtfoods, you've had great success, but it doesn't end now. While we do not advocate more restrictions on calories, your diet should still have enough Sirtfood. Many of our consumers are now at their ideal body shape continue to eat diets high in Sirtfood. The great thing about Sirtfoods is they are a lifestyle. In terms of weight management, the best way to think about them is that they help bring the body to the weight and composition it was intended to be. They work from here to preserve and hold you are looking great and feeling great. Essentially, this is the aim we wish for all adherents of the Sirtfood Diet.

9.   I have finished phase 2, so now should I stop drinking sirtfood green juice in the morning?

The green juice is our favorite way to start the day with a fantastic hit from Sirtfoods, so we endorse its long-term consumption. Our Sirtfood green juice has been carefully designed to include ingredients that provide a full spectrum of sirtuin-activating nutrients in potent dose-boosting fat-burning and wellness. We're all for variety, however, and while we recommend that you continue with a morning juice, we fully support anyone looking to experiment with various Sirtfood juice concoctions.

10. Are sirtfoods suitable for children?

The Sirtfood Diet is a powerful diet for weight loss and not intended for kids. That doesn't mean that kids should miss out on the excellent health benefits offered by including more Sirtfoods in their overall diet, though. For babies, a vast majority of Sirtfoods reflect incredibly healthy foods and help them achieve good and nutritious diets. Many of the meals planned for the diet's Phase 2 have been developed with families in mind, including the taste buds of babies. The likes of the Sirtfood pizza, the chili con carne, and the Sirtfood bites are perfect child-friendly foods with a nutritional value higher than usual children's food offerings. While most Sirtfoods are incredibly healthy for children to eat, the green juice that is too rich in fat-burning sirtfoods is not approved. We also advise against important caffeine sources, such as coffee and green tea. You will also need to be vigilant of chilies being included and may choose to keep things milder for kids.

11. Will I get any headache or feel tired during phase 1?

Phase 1 of the Sirtfood Diet offers strong naturally occurring food compounds in quantities that most people wouldn't get through their healthy diet, and some people will respond when they adjust to this drastic dietary shift. This may include symptoms such as mild headache or tiredness, although these effects are minor and short-lived in our experience. Of course, if the signs are serious or give you cause for concern, we suggest that you seek medical advice promptly. We have never seen anything other than occasional mild symptoms that quickly resolve, and within a few days, most people find that they have a renewed sense of energy, vigor, and well-being.

12. Should I take any supplements?

Unless your doctor or another health-care professional prescribe explicitly for you, we do not recommend indiscriminate use of nutritional supplements. You will be ingesting from Sirtfoods a vast and synergistic array of natural plant compounds, and it is these that will do you good. You cannot duplicate such benefits with nutritional supplements, and some nutritional supplements, such as antioxidants, can potentially conflict with the beneficial effects of Sirtfoods, which is the last thing you want, particularly if taken at high doses. Whenever possible, we think that getting the nutrients you need from eating a balanced diet rich in Sirtfoods is much better than taking the nutrients in the form of a pill. However, Vegans will have special nutritional considerations and our specific recommendations for those following diets which are purely plant-based. Furthermore, since plant proteins are lower in leucine, the amino acid that enhances Sirtfoods' actions, we have found that vegans can benefit from supplementing their diet with appropriate vegan protein powder. It refers in turn to those who perform high levels of exercise. This supplement should be taken off the Sirtfood green juice at a separate time of day.

13. Does the Sirtfood diet provide enough amount of fibers?

Many Sirtfoods are, of course, rich fibers. Onions, endive, and walnuts are popular examples, with buckwheat and Medjool dates mainly sticking out, suggesting the fiber department is not deprived of a Sirtfood-rich diet. Even in Phase 1, when food consumption is reduced, most of us will still consume the amount of fiber we're used to, especially if we select from the menu options the recipes that contain buckwheat, beans, and lentils. Nonetheless, for others reported to be vulnerable to intestinal problems such as constipation without higher intakes of fiber, an appropriate fiber supplement may be recommended during Phase 1, particularly Days 1 to 3, which should be addressed with your health care professional.

14. Is it mandatory to do phase 1 for seven days – can I do fewer?

There is nothing magical about seven days in Phase 1. Simply that is what we decided for our trial. We went for that because it was long enough to produce impressive results, but not long enough to make things arduous. It fits neatly into the lives of people as well. It was tested for seven days and what is proven to be effective. However, if you want to cut it short by a day or two for whatever reason, do so by completing until the end of Day 5 or Day 6. Don't worry, the lion's share of the benefits will still be reaped.

References

- Haigis, M. C., & Guarente, L. P. (2006). Mammalian sirtuins—emerging roles in physiology, aging, and calorie restriction. *Genes & development*, *20*(21), 2913-2921.
- Aragonès, G., Ardid-Ruiz, A., Ibars, M., Suárez, M., & Bladé, C. (2016). Modulation of leptin resistance by food compounds. *Molecular nutrition & food research*, *60*(8), 1789-1803.
- Ryall, J. G., Dell'Orso, S., Derfoul, A., Juan, A., Zare, H., Feng, X., ... & Sartorelli, V. (2015). The NAD+-dependent SIRT deacetylase translates a metabolic switch into regulatory epigenetics in skeletal muscle stem cells. *Cell stem cell*, *16*(2), 171-183.
- Wilking, M. J., & Ahmad, N. (2015). The role of SIRT in cancer: the saga continues. *The American journal of pathology*, *185*(1), 26.
- Si, H., & Liu, D. (2014). Dietary antiaging phytochemicals and mechanisms associated with prolonged survival. *The Journal of nutritional biochemistry*, *25*(6), 581-591.
- Duarte, D. A., Mariana Ap B, R., Papadimitriou, A., Silva, K. C., Amancio, V. H. O., Mendonça, J. N., ... & de Faria, J. M. L. (2015). Polyphenol-enriched cocoa protects the diabetic retina from glial reaction through the sirtuin pathway. *The Journal of nutritional biochemistry*, *26*(1), 64-74.
- Luccarini, I., Pantano, D., Nardiello, P., Cavone, L., Lapucci, A., Miceli, C., ... & Casamenti, F. (2016). The polyphenol oleuropein aglycone modulates the PARP1-SIRT interplay: an in vitro and in vivo study. *Journal of Alzheimer's Disease*, *54*(2), 737-750.
- Ibarrola-Jurado, N., Bulló, M., Guasch-Ferré, M., Ros, E., Martínez-González, M. A., Corella, D., ... & Arós, F. (2013).

Cross-sectional assessment of nut consumption and obesity, metabolic syndrome and other cardiometabolic risk factors: the PREDIMED study. *PloS one*, *8*(2).

- Yao, K., Duan, Y., Li, F., Tan, B., Hou, Y., Wu, G., & Yin, Y. (2016). Leucine in obesity: therapeutic prospects. *Trends in pharmacological sciences*, *37*(8), 714-727.
- Hosseini, A., & Hosseinzadeh, H. (2015). A review on the effects of Allium sativum (Garlic) in metabolic syndrome. *Journal of endocrinological investigation*, *38*(11), 1147-1157.
- Baliga, M. S., Baliga, B. R. V., Kandathil, S. M., Bhat, H. P., & Vayalil, P. K. (2011). A review of the chemistry and pharmacology of the date fruits (Phoenix dactylifera L.). *Food research international*, *44*(7), 1812-1822.
- Niseteo, T., Komes, D., Belščak-Cvitanović, A., Horžić, D., & Budeč, M. (2012). Bioactive composition and antioxidant potential of different commonly consumed coffee brews affected by their preparation technique and milk addition. *Food chemistry*, *134*(4), 1870-1877.
- Aune, D., Navarro Rosenblatt, D. A., Chan, D. S., Vieira, A. R., Vieira, R., Greenwood, D. C., ... & Norat, T. (2015). Dairy products, calcium, and prostate cancer risk: a systematic review and meta-analysis of cohort studies. *The American journal of clinical nutrition*, *101*(1), 87-117.
- Melnik, B. C. (2015). Milk—a nutrient system of mammalian evolution promoting mTORC1-dependent translation. *International journal of molecular sciences*, *16*(8), 17048-17087.

Sirtfood diet cookbook More than 80 healthy recipes to reset your metabolism and lose weight. Included a meal plan to start and get some results as soon as possible

CHAPTER ONE
WEEK AFTER WEEK DIET PROGRAM
Your feast organizer

This eating regimen depends on a two phase, three-week plan. Week one is a concentrated seven-day program intended to launch weight reduction.

Weeks two and three are a support plan intended for proceeded with weight reduction (expect around 1-2lbs every week) and better wellbeing.

Pick your feast decisions from the rundown underneath.

WEEK 1

Day 1 to 3 (1,000 calories for every day)

• Breakfast: Sirtfood green juice

• Mid-morning: Green juice

• Lunch: Green juice

• Dinner: Choice from underneath, in addition to 15–20g dull chocolate

Day 4 to 7 (1,500 calories for each day)

Plan as above, yet you drop one of the everyday green squeezes and supplant it with a second day by day supper – either a morning meal or lunch from the rundown underneath.

WEEKS 2 AND 3 (not calorie tallied)

Every day ought to include:

• 3 x sirtfood principle dinners

• 1 sirtfood green juice

- 2 snacks, browse a little bunch of pecans, strawberries or blueberries or an apple

Morning meals

- Green juice (see formula beneath)

- Sirtfood omelet – with bacon, parsley, chicory

- Greek yogurt – with 10g ground dim chocolate, slashed pecans and blended berries

- Spiced fried eggs – with bean stew and turmeric

Snacks

- Baked cod with sautéed greens

- Vegetable and kidney bean stew with prepared potato

- Waldorf plate of mixed greens with red onion, celery, apples and pecans

- Baked chicken bosom with pecan and parsley pesto and red onion plate of mixed greens

Suppers

- Prawn pan sear with buckwheat noodles (see formula underneath)

- Chicken bosom with tomato and stew salsa

- Salmon filet with chicory, rocket and celery plate of mixed greens

- Beef with red wine, onion rings and herb broiled potatoes (see formula underneath)

- Tuscan bean stew (see formula underneath)

Sirtfood green juice (Serves 1)

Purifying: Sirtfood green juice

2 enormous bunches (75g) kale

Enormous bunch (30g) rocket

Small bunch (5g) level leaf parsley

2–3 enormous stems (150g) green celery – including leaves

A large portion of a green apple

Juice of half lemon and half tsp matcha.

To make:

1.   Juice all the fixings aside from the green tea. At that point blend a modest quantity of juice in a glass with the matcha and mix vivaciously with a fork, at that point include the remainder of the juice to the glass and blend once more.

2.   You can make up the entirety of your juices for the day in one clump toward the beginning of the day, and refrigerate until required.

Prawn Stir-fry with Noodles (serves 1)

Sound: Prawn pan sear with noodles

- 150g shelled crude prawns

- 2 tsp soy sauce

- 2 tsp additional virgin olive oil

- 75g soba (buckwheat noodles)

- 1 cleaved garlic clove

- 1 cleaved superior stew

- 1 tsp finely cleaved new ginger

- 20g red onions - cut

- 40g celery, cut,

- 75g green beans - cleaved,

- 50g cleaved kale,

- 100ml chicken stock.

To make:

1.   Cook the prawns in a hot skillet with 1tsp of the soy and 1 tsp of the oil for 2 minutes and put to the other side. Cook the noodles as coordinated on the parcel. Channel and put in a safe spot.

2.   Meanwhile, fry flavors and veg in the rest of the oil over a medium–high warmth for 2–3 minutes. Add the stock and bring to the bubble, at that point stew for a moment or two, until the vegetables are cooked yet at the same time crunchy.

3.   Add the prawns and noodles to the dish, take back to the bubble. Expel from the warmth and serve.

Meat with red wine, onion rings and herb simmered potatoes (serves 1)

Healthy: Beef with red wine, onion rings and herb-simmered potatoes

- 100g potatoes - stripped and cut into 2cm pieces

- 1 tbsp additional virgin olive oil

- 5g parsley - finely slashed

- 50g red onion-cut into rings

- 50g cut kale

- 1 garlic clove - finely slashed

- 150g hamburger steak

- 40ml red wine

- 150ml hamburger stock

- 1 tsp tomato purée

- 1 tsp corn flour - disintegrated in 1 tbsp water

To make:

1. Heat the broiler to 220C/gas 7. Heat up the potatoes for 5 minutes, at that point channel. Spot in a simmering tin with 1 tsp of the oil and dish for 35–45 minutes. Turn at regular intervals. At the point when cooked, evacuate, sprinkle with the cleaved parsley and blend well.

2. Fry onion in 1 tsp of the oil over a medium warmth for 5–7 minutes, until pleasantly caramelized. Steam the kale for 2–3 minutes at that point channel. Fry the garlic delicately in ½ teaspoon of oil for 1 moment, until delicate, include the kale and fry for a further 1–2 minutes, until delicate.

3. Coat the hamburger with ½ a teaspoon of the oil and fry in a hot container over a medium warmth, as per how you like it cooked. Expel from the skillet and put aside to rest.

4. Add the wine to the hot skillet and decrease significantly, until sweet. Include the stock and tomato purée and bring to the bubble, at that point add the corn flour glue to thicken, a little at once. Serve hamburger with broil potatoes, kale, onion rings and red wine sauce.

Tuscan bean stew (Serves 1)

Taste of Italy: Tuscan Bean Stew

1 tbsp additional virgin olive oil

50g red onion, finely cleaved 30g carrot, finely hacked 30g celery, finely slashed

1 garlic clove, finely cleaved

1 tsp herbs de Provence 200ml vegetable stock

1 x 400g tin cleaved tomatoes 1 tsp tomato puree

200g tinned blended beans

50g kale, cleaved

138208672551

1 tbsp cleaved parsley

40g buckwheat to serve

To make:

1.   Heat oil in a pot over a low–medium warmth and tenderly fry the onion, carrot, celery, garlic and herbs, until the veg are delicate.

2.   Add the stock, tomatoes and tomato puree and bring to the bubble. Include the beans and stew for 30 minutes. Include the kale and cook for another 5–10 minutes, until delicate, at that point include the parsley.

3.   Cook the buckwheat as indicated by parcel guidelines, channel and serve.

The best technique to Meal Prep You Week of Meals:

1.   Make a gathering of the Vegan Pancakes to have for breakfast on Days 1, 5 and 7. Store the cooked hotcakes in a singular layer in a water/air confirmation holder harden until arranged to eat; warm in the microwave.

2.   Cook a gathering of Basic Quinoa to have for lunch on Day 2 and dinner on Day 5.

3.   Make the Quinoa and Chia Oatmeal Mix to have on Day 4. Store the dry mix in an invulnerable holder for whatever length of time that multi month.

Day 1

Breakfast (296 calories)

- 2 Vegan Pancakes

- 1/4 cup blackberries

- 1 Tbsp. nutty spread

Mix nutty spread in with 1 tsp. warm water (or increasingly, fluctuating, to scatter the nutty spread). Sprinkle over hotcakes.

A.M. Chomp (150 calories)

- 3/4 cup edamame units, arranged with a dash of salt

Lunch (245 calories)

- 1 serving White Bean and Avocado Toast

- 1 cup cut cucumber

P.M. Chomp (30 calories)

- 1 little plum

Dinner (499 calories)

- 1 serving Falafel Salad with Lemon-Tahini Dressing

Step by step Totals: 1,221 calories, 50 g protein, 137 g starches, 38 g fiber, 59 g fat, 1,586 mg sodium

Day 2

Breakfast (262 calories)

- 1 serving Peanut Butter and Chia Berry Jam English Muffin

A.M. Chomp (100 calories)

- 1/2 cup edamame units, arranged with a pinch of salt

Lunch (360 calories)

- 4 cups White Bean and Veggie Salad

In the event that you're taking this plate of blended greens to go, get it together in this advantageous dining experience prep compartment, unequivocally made to keep your greens new and dressing separate until you're set up to eat.

Dinner (500 calories)

- 2 cups Black-Bean Quinoa Buddha Bowl

Step by step Totals: 1,220 calories, 48 g protein, 153 g starches, 46 g fiber, 53 g fat, 1,370 mg sodium

Day 3

Breakfast (266 calories)

- 1 serving Peanut Butter-Banana Toast

A.M. Goody (114 calories)

- 2 Tbsp. pumpkin seeds (pepitas)

Lunch (325 calories)

- 4 cups serving Green Salad with Edamame and Beets

P.M. Goody (62 calories)

- 2 cups air-popped popcorn

Dinner (446 calories)

- 1 1/2 cups Roasted Cauliflower and Potato Curry Soup
- 1/2 minimal whole wheat pita, toasted

- 1/3 cup hummus

Banquet Prep Tip: Save 1 serving of the Roasted Cauliflower and Potato Curry Soup in a watertight supper prep holder for lunch on Day 4.

Step by step Totals: 1,213 calories, 49 g protein, 132 g starches, 34 g fiber, 57 g fat, 1,760 mg sodium

Day 4

Breakfast (296 calories)

- 1/3 cup Quinoa and Chia Oatmeal Mix cooked with 1/4 cups unsweetened soymilk

Banquet Prep Tip: Make the Quinoa and Chia Oatmeal Mix and store in a fixed shut compartment for whatever length of time that multi month.

A.M. Goody (30 calories)

- 1 little plum

Lunch (309 calories)

- 1 1/2 cups Roasted Cauliflower and Potato Curry Soup

- 1/2 minimal whole wheat pita, toasted

P.M. Goody (114 calories)

- 2 Tbsp. pumpkin seeds (pepitas)

Dinner (472 calories)

- 1 serving Stuffed Sweet Potato with Hummus Dressing

Step by step Totals: 1,222 calories, 51 g protein, 177 g starches, 40 g fiber, 40 g fat, 1,327 mg sodium

Day 5

Breakfast (296 calories)

- 2 Vegan Pancakes

- 1/4 cup blackberries

- 1 Tbsp. nutty spread

Mix nutty spread in with 1 tsp. warm water (or progressively, changing, to scatter the nutty spread). Sprinkle over hotcakes.

Lunch (325 calories)

- 1 serving Veggie and Hummus Sandwich

P.M. Chomp (100 calories)

- 1/2 cup edamame units, arranged with a bit of salt

Dinner (487 calories)

- 1 cup Chickpea Curry

- 1 cup Basic Quinoa

Step by step Totals: 1,208 calories, 44 g protein, 149 g starches, 33 g fiber, 50 g fat, 1,253 mg sodium

Day 6

Breakfast (262 calories)

- 1 serving Peanut Butter and Chia Berry Jam English Muffin

A.M. Nibble (17 calories)

- 1/4 cup hummus

- 2 medium celery stems, cut into sticks

Lunch (308 calories)

- 1 serving Vegan Bistro Lunch Box

- 2 Tbsp. pumpkin seeds (pepitas)

Dinner (525 calories)

- 1 serving Thai Spaghetti Squash with Peanut Sauce

- 1 cup Vegan Thai Cucumber Salad

Step by step Totals: 1,211 calories, 51 g protein, 118 g sugars, 32 g fiber, 65 g fat, 2,065 mg sodium

Day 7

Breakfast (296 calories)

- 2 Vegan Pancakes

- 1/4 cup blackberries

- 1 Tbsp. nutty spread

Mix nutty spread in with 1 tsp. warm water (or progressively, differing, to scatter the nutty spread). Sprinkle over pancakes.

A.M. Goody (62 calories)

- 1 medium orange

Lunch (325 calories)

- 4 cups serving Green Salad with Edamame and Beets

P.M. Goody (93 calories)

- 3 cups air-popped popcorn

Dinner (434 calories)

- 1 serving Rainbow Veggie Spring Roll Bowl

Step by step Totals: 1,209 calories, 45 g protein, 144 g sugars, 32 g fiber, 51 g fat, 1,732 mg sodium

You Did It!

Well done on finishing this veggie darling weight decrease supper plan. Perhaps you followed every single supper and snack or possibly just used it as an influential guide for following a veggie darling eating regimen. Regardless, we believe you found this course of action fascinating, delightful and edifying. Following a plant-based having routine supper plan is a sound technique to get fit as a fiddle and keep it off. Continue doing magnificent one of our other sound veggie sweetheart supper plans or vegetarian feast plans.

Alongside this fat-consuming impact, sirtfoods likewise have the exceptional capacity to -naturally control craving and increment muscle work – making them the ideal answer for accomplishing a sound weight.

Without a doubt, their wellbeing boosting impacts are ground-breaking to such an extent that a few examinations have demonstrated them to be more viable than physician endorsed sedates in forestalling ceaseless ailment, with evident -benefits in diabetes, coronary illness and -Alzheimer's infection.

No big surprise societies eating the most sirtfoods – including Japan and Italy – are the least fatty and most beneficial on the planet. What's more, that is the reason we've contrived an eating regimen based around them.

The sirtfood list

Sirtfoods are for the most part promptly accessible and -accessible nourishments. The most powerful ones include: red wine, dull chocolate, dark espresso, kale, rocket, parsley, red onions, strawberries, pecans, additional virgin olive oil, curry flavors, green tea, blueberries, celery, bean stew, apples and buckwheat.

What's the proof?

We trialed our eating regimen at a rec center in South West London, basically to test and improve wellbeing. We were shocked by the outcomes. Members normally lost 7lbs in seven days, and saw increments in bulk, prosperity and vitality.

We anticipated that individuals should lose some weight yet never foreseen that it would be so a lot, nor that individuals would keep up or even increase some muscle, which is uncommon when slimming down.

CHAPTER TWO
The Sirte Food Recipes
TURMERIC CHICKEN & KALE SALAD WITH Honey-lime DRESSING-SIRTFOOD RECIPES

Prep-time

20 moment

Prepare moment

10 moment

Complete time

Thirty moment

Notes: When planning beforehand, dress the salad 10 minutes earlier Functioning. Chicken might be substituted with beef chopped, sliced prawns or fish. Vegetarians may use chopped cooked or mushrooms quinoa.

Serves: two

Substances

For your poultry

* 1) tsp ghee or one tablespoon coconut-oil

* 1/2 moderate brown onion, diced

* 250 300 grams / 9 ounces. Chicken mince or chopped chicken up eyebrow

* 1 large garlic clove, finely grated

* inch tsp peppermint powder

* 1teaspoon lime zest

1 teaspoon of 1/2 carrot

* 1/2 tsp salt

For your salad

* 6 broccoli 2 or two glasses of broccoli florets

* two tablespoon pumpkin seeds (pepitas)

* 3 substantial kale leaves, stalks removed and sliced

* 1/2 avocado, chopped

* bunch of coriander leaves, sliced

* bunch of fresh mint leaves, sliced

For your dressing table

* 3 tablespoon carrot juice

* 1 small garlic clove, finely diced or grated

* 3 tablespoon teaspoons Coconut Oil (I used 1 teaspoon tablespoon coconut and 2 tablespoon EVO)

1 tsp raw honey

* 1/2 tsp Whole-grain or Dijon chopped

* 1/2 tsp sea pepper and salt

Guidelines

Inch. Heat the ghee or coconut oil at a tiny skillet on tepid to warm. Insert the onion and then sauté on moderate heat for 45 minutes, till gold. Insert the chicken blossom and garlic and simmer for 2 3 minutes on medium-high warmth, breaking it all out.

2. Insert the garlic, lime zest, lime juice, pepper and salt and cook stirring often, to get a further 34 minutes. Place the cooked toaster apart.

3. As the chicken is cooking, bring a little bit of water. Insert the broccolini and prepare 2 weeks. Wipe warm water and then dip into 3-4 pieces every.

4. Insert the pumpkin seeds into the skillet out of the toast and chicken over moderate heat for two minutes, stirring often to avoid burning off. Year with just a tiny bit of salt. Establish a side. Raw pumpkin seeds will also be nice tousle.

5. Put chopped spinach at a salad bowl and then pour the dressing table. Together with your fingers, massage and toss the carrot with all your dressing table. This may dampen the lettuce, sort of just like exactly what citrus fruit will not steak or fish carpaccio -- it 'hamburgers' it marginally.

6. Eventually throw throughout the cooked poultry, broccoli, refreshing blossoms, pumpkin seeds and avocado pieces.

BUCKWHEAT NOODLES WITH CHICKEN KALE & MISO DRESSING-SIRTFOOD RECIPES

Prep time: 15 mins Cook time: 15 mins Absolute time: 30 mins

1: two

Elements

for Those noodles

* 2 3 handfuls of kale leaves (eliminated in the stem along with approximately sliced)

* 150 grams / 5-ounce buckwheat noodles (100 percent buckwheat (no wheat)

* 34 shiitake mushrooms, chopped

* 1 tsp coconut oil or ghee

* 1) brown onion, finely manicured

* Inch moderate sized poultry breast, chopped or grated

* 1 red chili, thinly chopped (seeds directly or outside based on just how hot you really like it)

* two large garlic cloves, finely manicured

* 23 tablespoon Tamari sauce (fermented soy sauce)

For your own miso dressing

* Inch 1/2 tablespoon New Natural miso

* 1) tablespoon Tamari sauce

* 1) tablespoon teaspoon Essential Olive Oil

* 1 tablespoon lime or lemon juice

1 tsp coconut oil (discretionary)

Guidelines

Inch. Provide a medium saucepan of water. Insert the carrot and cook 1 minute, until slightly wilted. Take out and place a side but book the drinking water and also make back it into the boil. Insert the soba noodles and cook in line with the package guidelines (commonly roughly five min). Wipe warm water and also place a side.

2. At the interim, pan presses the shiitake mushrooms at just a tiny ghee or coconut oil (approximately a tsp) to get 2 3 minutes, till lightly browned on each individual facet. Sprinkle with sea salt and then place a side.

3. At precisely the exact skillet, warm coconut oil or ghee more than medium-high warmth. Sauté onion and simmer for 2 3 minutes then add the chicken bits. Cook 5 minutes on moderate heat, stirring a handful times, you can put in the garlic, tamari sauce as well as only a bit of dab of plain water. Prepare for a further 2-3 minutes, stirring often until salmon is cooked through.

4. At length, insert the carrot and soba noodles and then chuck throughout the chicken to heat upward.

5. Mix that the miso dressing table and scatter across the noodles directly at the conclusion of ingestion this fashion in which you can retain dozens of enzymes that are beneficial at the miso living and busy.

ASIAN KING PRAWN Stir Fry WITH BUCKWHEAT NOODLES -- SIRTFOOD RECIPES

Serves Inch

Elements:

150g shelled raw king prawns, deveined

two tsp tamari (it's possible to utilize soy sauce in the event that you aren't keeping away from gluten)

two teaspoon extra virgin coconut oil

75g soba (buckwheat noodles)

inch tsp clove, finely chopped

inch hen's eye chili, finely chopped

inch teaspoon finely chopped fresh ginger

20g red onions, chopped

40g celery, trimmed and chopped

75g green beans, sliced

50g lettuce, approximately sliced

100ml poultry inventory

5g lovage or celery leaves Instructions:

Heat a skillet on a high temperature, cook the prawns into 1 tsp of this tamari plus one tsp of this oil to two --three full minutes. Transfer the prawns into an individual plate. Wipe out the pan using kitchen paper, even since you are definitely going to utilize it.

Prepare the noodles in warm water 58 minutes as directed on the package. Drain and place a side.

Meanwhile, fry the garlic, peppermint and eucalyptus, red celery, onion, legumes and lettuce at the rest of the oil over a moderate -- higher temperature for two --three full minutes. Insert the stock and bring to the boil and simmer for an instant or 2, before veggies have been cooked but still crispy.

Insert the prawns, noodles and then lovage/celery leaves into the pan, then return to the boil and then remove from heat and function.

BAKED SALMON SALAD WITH CREAMY MINT DRESSING-SIRTFOOD RECIPES

340 Energy • 3 your SIRT 5 per day

Baking the salmon at the oven creates this salad really easy.

Serves Inch • All Set at 20 moments

1) salmon fillet (130g)

40g Combined salad renders

40g youthful lettuce leaves

two radishes, trimmed and finely chopped

5cm slice (50g) lettuce, cut chunks

Two spring onions, trimmed and chopped

Inch little couple (10g) parsley, roughly sliced

For your dressing table:

Inch teaspoon low-carb turkey

Inch tablespoon organic yogurt

Inch tablespoon rice

2 renders mint, finely chopped

Salt and freshly milled black pepper

1) Preheat the oven to 200°C (one hundred eighty °C fan/Gas 6).

Two Position the carrot wedges onto the baking dish and bake for 16--18 minutes before cooked. Remove from the oven and place a side. The salmon is every bit as fine cold or hot within the salad. If a poultry contains skin, then just brush down skin and clear away the salmon out of skin by means of a fish piece after ingestion. It will slide easily once cooked.

3 At a little bowl mix together the mayonnaise, yogurt, rice vinegar, mint leaves and pepper and salt together and make to endure five or more minutes to permit the

tastes to grow.

4 Order the salad lettuce and leaves onto the serving plate and top together with all the radishes, celery, celery, spring onions and skillet. Flake the carrot on the salad and then drizzle the dressing.

Choc-chip GRANOLA-SIRTFOOD RECIPES

244 Energy

1/2 your SIRT 5 per day

Coffee! Make sure you Work using a cup of green tea extract to supply you with lots of SIRTs. The rice malt syrup might be substituted with walnut syrup should you would like.

Serves 8 • All Set at Half an Hour

200g jumbo oats

50g pecans, approximately

sliced

3 tablespoons mild olive oil

20g butter

Inch tablespoon dark brown sugar

Two tablespoon rice malt g

60g high quality (70 percent)

black chocolate chips

1) Preheat the oven to 160°C (One Hundred Forty °C fan/Gas 3). Line a large baking dish having a silicone sheet or baking parchment.

Two Blend the oats and pecans collectively at a big bowl. At a modest skillet, lightly warm the coconut oil, butter, brown rice and sugar malt butter before butter has melted and the sugar and butter consumed simmer. Usually do not let it boil. Pour the syrup on the ginger and stir completely before the oats are wholly coated.

3 Fragrant the granola within the baking Menu, dispersing into the corners. Go away clumps of mix using dimension as opposed to an additional disperse. Bake in the oven for about 20 minutes before only pops gold brown at the borders. Remove from the oven and then leave to cool to the menu altogether.

4 Once cool, divide some larger Lumps about the plate together along with your palms and mix in the chocolate chips. Twist or put the granola in an air-tight jar or tub. The granola will continue for a minimum of two months.

Aromatic ASIAN HOTPOT-SIRTFOOD RECIPES

185 Energy

1 1/2 of you personally SIRT 5 per day

Serves 2 • All Set at 1-5 moments

1 teaspoon tomato purée

Inch star anise, crushed (or 1/4 tsp ground anise)

Modest handful (10g) parsley, stalks finely chopped

Modest couple (1Og) coriander, stalks finely chopped

Juice of 1/2 lime

500ml chicken stock, fresh or produced using Inch block

1/2 lettuce, peeled and cut into matchsticks

50g lettuce, cut into small florets

50g beansprouts

1OOg raw tiger prawns

1OOg Organization broccoli, sliced

50g rice noodles, cooked according to packet directions

50g cooked Drinking Water chestnuts, emptied

20g sushi ginger, sliced

Inch tablespoon high miso glue

Set the tomato purée, celebrity anise, parsley stalks, coriander pops, carrot Juice and chicken stock in a huge pan and bring to a simmer for about 10 seconds.

Insert the lettuce, lettuce, prawns, tofu, noodles and water chestnuts along with Simmer lightly till the prawns are cooked through. Remove from heat and stir from the ice ginger and also miso paste.

Drink sprinkled with the coriander and parsley leaves.

LAMB, Butternut squash AND Day TAGINE-SIRTFOOD RECIPES

Prep-time

1-5 mins

Cook moment

Inch hour 15 mins

Complete period

Inch hour 30 mins

Extraordinary warming Moroccan spices Create this nutritious tagine ideal for cold autumn and chilly evenings. Drink buckwheat to get an excess wellness kick!

Serves: 4

Substances

2 tablespoon olive oil

1) red onion, sliced

2cm ginger, grated

3 tsp cloves, grated or smashed

Inch tsp chili flakes (or to taste)

2 tsp cumin seeds

1 teaspoon cinnamon stick

2 tsp ground turmeric

800g lamb neck fillet, cut into 2cm balls

1/2 tsp salt

100g Medrol dates, pitted and sliced

400g tin chopped berries, and half a can of plain water

500g butternut chopped chopped into 1cm cubes

400g tin Chick Peas, emptied

2 tablespoon fresh coriander (and additional for garnish)

Buckwheat, Cous-cous, Flat Breads or corn to function

Method

Inch. Pre heat your oven to 140C.

2. Drizzle about two tablespoon of coconut oil in to a large oven proof sauce pan or throw iron dish dish. Insert the chopped onion and then cook over a gentle heat, together with the lid for around five minutes, before the onions are softened but not too brown.

3. Insert the grated ginger and garlic, chili, cumin, cinnamon, and garlic. Stir very well and cook 1 minute with all off the lid. Insert a dash of water when it becomes overly tender.

4. Next insert from the carrot balls. Stir to coat the beef from the spices and onions and add the salt chopped meats and berries, and roughly half of a can of plain water (100-200ml).

5. B ring the tagine into the boil and then put the lid and place on your skillet for about 1 hour and a quarter hour.

6. Ten minutes prior to the conclusion of this cooking period, include the chopped butternut squash and emptied chickpeas. Stir everything

together, set the lid on and come back to the oven to the last half an hour of ingestion.

7. After the tagine is able to remove from the oven and then stir fry the sliced coriander. Drink buckwheat, cous-cous, flat breads or basmati rice.

Notes

In the Event You do not Have an ovenproof spade or throw iron dish dish, just cook That the tagine at a normal spout up till it must proceed from the oven and then Move the tagine to a routine lidded casserole dish ahead of setting from the oven. Insert in an Additional Five minutes cooking period Allowing to the Simple Fact the Casserole dish will probably be needing added time for you to warm up.

PRAWN ARRABBIATA-SIRTFOOD RECIPES

Serves Inch

Preparing time:

3-5 -- Forty moments

Cooking moment:

20 -- Thirty moments

Ingredients

125-150 g Bite or cooked prawns (Preferably king prawns)

Sixty-Five-gram Buckwheat pasta

Inch tablespoon Extra virgin coconut oil

To get arrabbiata sauce

Forty grams Crimson onion, finely chopped

1 teaspoon Garlic clove, finely chopped

Thirty-gram Celery, finely chopped

Inch Bird's-eye peeled, finely chopped

Inch teaspoon grated mixed veggies

Inch teaspoon Extra virgin Coconut Oil

Two tablespoon White wine (discretionary)

Four Hundred grams Tinned chopped berries

Inch tablespoon Chopped parsley

Method

Inch. Stir the garlic, onion, celery along with peppermint and peppermint blossoms at the oil over a moderate --low-heat for 1--two weeks. Turn up the heat to moderate, bring the wine and cook 1 second. Insert the berries and also leave the sauce simmer past a moderate --reduced heat for 20--half an hour, before it's a wonderful rich texture. In the event you're feeling that the sauce is still becoming overly thick only put in just a tiny H2o.

2. As the sauce is cooking attract a bowl of water into the boil and then cook the pasta in line with the package directions. When cooked to your dish, drain, then toss with the coconut oil and also maintain from the pan before essential.

3. If you're employing uncooked prawns put them into the sauce and then cook for a further 3--4 minutes, then till they've turned opaque and pink then put in the skillet and function. If you're employing cooked prawns insert them using all the skillet, then bring the sauce to the boil and then function.

4. Insert the cooked pasta into the sauce, then combine thoroughly but lightly and function.

TURMERIC BAKED SALMON-SIRTFOOD RECIPES

Serves: 1)

Preparing time:

10 -- 1-5 moments

Cooking moment:

10 moments

Ingredients

125-150 gram Skinned Salmon

Inch teaspoon Extra virgin olive oil oil

Inch teaspoon Ground turmeric

1/4 Juice with the lemon

For your hot carrot

Inch teaspoon Extra virgin Coconut Oil

Forty grams Red onion, finely chopped

Sixty grams Tinned green peas

1 teaspoon Garlic clove, finely chopped

Inch tsp fresh ginger, finely chopped

1 teaspoon Bird's eye peeled, finely chopped

150 grams Celery, cut into 2cm lengths

Inch teaspoon moderate Curry-powder

130-gram Tomato, cut into eight wedges

100 M L vegetable or pasta inventory

Inch tablespoon Chopped parsley

Method

Heat the oven to 200C / gas mark 6.

2 focus on the hot celery. Heat a skillet above a moderate --reduced heat, then add the coconut oil, then and then a garlic, onion, ginger, chili, and celery. Fry lightly for two --three minutes until softened but not colored, you can put in the curry powder and cook for a more moment.

Insert the berries subsequently your lentils and stock and simmer for 10 minutes. You might need to raise or reduce the cooking period according to what lean you'd like your own sausage.

Meanwhile, blend the garlic oil and lemon juice and then rub the salmon. # Set on the skillet and cook 8--10 seconds.

in order to complete, stir the skillet throughout the sausage and then function with all the salmon.

CHAPTER THREE
SALAD-SIRTFOOD RECIPES

Serves Inch

Planning time: 5 minutes

Ingredients

75 grams Natural Steak

Juice of 1/4 using the lemon

Inch teaspoon Coriander, sliced

Inch teaspoon Ground turmeric

1/2 tsp moderate Curry-powder

One Hundred g Cooked Chicken, cut to bite-sized Parts

6 Walnut pliers, finely chopped

1 teaspoon Medjool Day, finely chopped

20 grams Crimson pumpkin, diced

Inch loaf's eye chili

Forty-gram Rocket, to function

Method

Blend the lemon, lemon juice, spices and coriander together in a bowl. Insert each of the ingredients and serve over the mattress of this rocket.

BAKED POTATOES WITH SPICY Chick-pea STEW-SIRTFOOD RECIPES

Prep-time

10 mins

Prepare moment

Inch hour

Serves 4 6

Kind of all Mexican Mole matches North African Tagine, this Spicy Chickpea Stew is Really yummy and leaves a fantastic topping for baked potatoes, also it merely appears to become vegan, vegan, gluten free and dairy. Plus, it comprises chocolate.

Ingredients

4 6 celery, pricked around

2 tablespoon coconut oil

2 red onions, finely chopped

4 tsp garlic, grated or smashed

2cm ginger, grated

1/2 -2 tsp teaspoons tablespoons (based how sexy you prefer matters)

2 tablespoon cumin seeds

2 tablespoon garlic

loaf of plain water

2 x 400g tins chopped berries

2 tablespoon unsweetened cocoa powder (or cacao)

2 x 400g tins chick peas (or kidney beans should you want) containing the chick-pea water do not DRAIN!!

Two yellow peppers (or anything color you would like!)), sliced into bitesize bits

2 tablespoon sliced and additional for garnish

Salt and pepper to taste (discretionary)

Facet salad (discretionary)

Method

Inch. Pre heat the oven to 200C, however it's possible to prepare all of your own ingredients.

2. After the oven is still sexy enough to put your baking potatoes from the oven and then cook for 1 hour until they do the way you prefer them.

3. As soon as the sausage come from the oven, set the coconut oil and sliced red onion into a large wide saucepan and cook lightly, together with the lid for five full minutes, then till the onions are tender but not too brown.

4. Remove the lid and then insert the ginger, garlic, cumin and simmer. Prepare for a more moment on the very low heat, you can add the garlic plus an exact compact·dab of warm water and then prepare for an additional moment, just take good care never to permit the pan get overly tender.

5. Then include the berries, cocoa powder (or even cacao), chick peas (which include the chick-pea h2o) and yellowish pepper.) Bring to the boil, and then simmer over a very low heat for 4-5 seconds before sauce is thick and unctuous (but do not allow it burn up). The stew ought to be performed at the exact same period whilst the legumes.

6. Ultimately stir at the two tablespoons of parsley, plus a few pepper and salt should you want, also function the stew in addition to the chopped sausage, possibly having an easy salad.

GRAPE AND MELON JUICE-SIRTFOOD RECIPES

125 Energy

2 your SIRT 5 a-day

Serves inch • all set in two minutes

1/2 pineapple, pared if chosen, halved, seeds removed and roughly sliced

30g youthful lettuce leaves, stalks eliminated

100g red seedless grapes

100g cantaloupe melon, peeled, deseeded and cut into balls

inch Combine together into a blender or juicer until clean.

KALE AND RED ONION DHAL WITH BUCKWHEAT-SIRTFOOD RECIPES

Prep-time

5 mins

Prepare moment

25 mins

Complete time

Thirty mins

Serves:4

Delectable and incredibly healthy that this Kale and Red Onion Dhal using Buckwheat is fast and simple to generate and normally gluten free, dairy free, vegetarian and vegetarian.

INGREDIENTS

1 tablespoon olive oil

1 small red onion, sliced

3 garlic cloves, grated or smashed

two tsp ginger, grated

inch birds-eye chili, deseeded and chopped (more if you prefer things sexy!)

2 tsp turmeric

2 tsp garam masala

160g reddish peas

400ml Coconut-milk

200ml H2o

100g lettuce (or lettuce are an Amazing choice)

160g buckwheat (or brown rice instead)

METHOD

Inch. Set the coconut oil into a sizable, deep skillet and put in the chopped onion. Cook on a minimal heat, together with the lid for five minutes until softened.

2. Insert the ginger, garlic and simmer and cook 1 minute.

3. Insert the garlic, garam masala and also a dash of drinking water and then cook for 1 minute.

4. Insert the red peas, almond milk, also 200ml drinking water (try so only by 50 percent of filling the coconut-milk may using plain water and stirring it in the saucepan).

5. Combine everything together completely and then cook 20 minutes over a lightly heat with the lid. Stir from time to time and add slightly bit more water in the event the dhal commences to stand.

6. After 20 seconds add the carrot, stir completely and then replace the lid, then prepare for a further five minutes (1 2 minutes in the event that you employ spinach)

7. Approximately fifteen seconds ahead of the curry is prepared, set the buckwheat at a medium sauce pan and then put in loads of warm H2o. Bring back the water into the boil and then cook for 10 minutes (or only a very little longer in the event that you would rather your buckwheat softer. Drain the buckwheat at a sieve and function using all the dhal.

Char-grilled BEEF WITH A RED WINE JUS, ONION RINGS, GARLIC KALE AND HERB ROASTED POTATOES-SIRTFOOD RECIPES

Elements:

100g celery, peeled and cut into 2cm Wars

Inch tablespoon extra-virgin Coconut Oil

5g tsp, finely chopped

50g red onion, chopped into circles

50g lettuce, chopped

Inch tsp clove, finely chopped

120--150g x ray 3.5cm-thick beef noodle beef or 2cm-thick sirloin beef

40ml reddish wine

150ml beef inventory

Inch teaspoon tomato purée

Inch teaspoon corn flour, dissolved in 1 tablespoon water

Guidelines:

Heat the oven to 220°C/petrol.

Put the sausage into a spoonful of boiling water, then return to the boil and then cook --5 minutes, then empty. Put into a skillet with 1 tsp of this oil and then roast at the oven for 3-5 --4-5 minutes. Twist the berries each 10 minutes to assure even cooking. After cooked, then remove from the oven, then scatter the skillet and combine nicely.

Fry the onion 1 tsp of the oil over a moderate heat for 5 minutes minutes, Until tender and well caramelized. Maintain heat. Steam the kale for two --three minutes then empty. Stir the garlic lightly in 1/2 tsp of petroleum for 1 minute, till tender but not colored. Insert the carrot and simmer for a further inch --two minutes, till tender. Maintain heat.

Heat an oven proof skillet on a high heat. Coat the beef in 1/2 a tsp of this oil and then stir from the popular pan above a moderate --high-heat depending on just how you would like your beef done. If you prefer your own beef moderate it'd be more straightforward to sear the beef and also transfer the pan into a toaster place in 220°C/petrol 7 and then complete the cooking which manner to your prescribed intervals.

Take out the beef in the pan and then reserve to break. Insert Your Wine into your sexy Pan to create any meat up deposit. Bubble to decrease your wine by half an hour an hour until syrupy along using a flavor that is concentrated.

Insert the tomato and stock purée into the beef pan and then bring to the boil, then then Insert the corn flour paste to thicken your sauce, so giving it only a very little at the same time and soon you've got your preferred consistency. Stir in all those juices out of the dinner that is rested and serve with the roasted lettuce, celery, onion bands and green berry sauce.

KALE AND Black-currant SMOOTHIE-SIRTFOOD RECIPES

86 Energy

Inch -- 1/2 of One's SIRT 5 per day

Serves 2 • All Set in 3 moments

2 teaspoon honey

1) cup freshly produced Green-tea

10 infant spinach leaves, stalks eliminated

Inch ripe banana

Forty gram blackcurrants, washed and stalks eliminated

6 Ice-cubes

Stir the honey in to the green Tea till simmer. Whiz each of the components together in a blender till smooth. Drink instantly.

BUCKWHEAT PASTA SALAD-SIRTFOOD RECIPES

Serves Inch

50g buckwheat pasta (cooked in Line with the package directions)

Sizable few rocket

Small number of basil leaves

8 cherry tomatoes, halved

1/2 avocado, coriander

10 tsp

inch tablespoon extra-virgin coconut oil

20g walnut nuts

Gradually combine all of the ingredients apart from the pine nuts and then arrange onto the plate or within a bowl, then then scatter the pine nuts on surface.

GREEK SALAD SKEWERS-SIRTFOOD RECIPES

306 Energy • 3.5 of One's SIRT 5 per day

Serves 2 • All Set at 10 moments

2 wooden skewers, soaked in plain water for 30 minutes earlier Utilize

8 big black olives

8 cherry tomatoes

1 yellow pepper, cut into 8 squares

1/2 reddish onion, then cut and separated to 8 bits

100g (roughly 10cm) cucumber, cut into 4 pieces and simmer

100g feta, cut into 8 cubes

For Your dressing:

1 tablespoon extra-virgin olive oil

Taste of 1/2 lemon

1 teaspoon balsamic vinegar

1/2 teaspoons garlic, crushed and peeled

Handful of leaves basil, finely chopped (or even 1/2 teaspoon dried blended Herbaceous plants to displace peppermint and eucalyptus)

Handful of leaves eucalyptus, thinly sliced

Generous flavor of salt and freshly ground black pepper

Inch tsp each skewer using all the salad components at the Order: tomato, olive, yellow pepper, red onion, cucumber, feta, olive, tomato oil, yellow pepper, red onion, cucumber, feta.

2 Put all of the dressing ingredients in a Little bowl and then blend Together completely. Pour the skewers.

KALE, EDAMAME AND to Fu CURRY-SIRTFOOD RECIPES

342 Energy

Two 1/2 your SIRT 5 per day

A heating and wintry curry. Simple to Keep possibly refrigerated or suspended for still another day.

Serves 4 • All Set at 4-5 minutes

Inch tablespoon rapeseed oil

1 big onion, sliced

4 tsp garlic, grated and peeled

Inch big thumb (7cm) fresh ginger, grated and peeled

Inch red chili, deseeded and finely chopped

1/2 tsp ground garlic

1/4 tsp Pepper

Inch teaspoon paprika

1/2 tsp ground cumin

Inch teaspoon salt

250g dried red peas

Inch liter hot water

50g frozen soya edamame legumes

200g Company carrot, sliced into cubes

2 tablespoons, roughly sliced

tsp of 1 tsp

200g lettuce leaves, stalks removed and ripped

Inch Set the oil at a heavy-bottomed pan on a low-medium warmth. Insert the onion and cook 5 min just before adding the ginger, garlic and simmer and ingestion for a further two minutes. Insert the garlic, cayenne, paprika, cumin and salt. Hurry before adding that the red peas and stirring.

Two Pour from the skillet and then bring about a simmer for about 10 minutes, then lower heat and cook for a further 20-30 minutes before curry includes a thick Porridge' consistency.

3 Insert the soya legumes, tomatoes and kale and then cook for a further five minutes. Insert the carrot juice and also kale leaves and then cook until the acidity isn't merely tender.

CHOCOLATE CUPCAKES WITH MATCHA ICING-SIRTFOOD RECIPES

2 3 4 Energy • Inch of One's SIRT 5 per cent Afternoon

Only magnificent!

MAKES 1-2 • All Set IN 3-5 MINUTES

150g self-rising flour

200g caster sugar

60g cocoa

1/2 teaspoon salt

1/2 teaspoon nice java coffee, decaf in case Favored

120ml milk

1/2 tsp vanilla infusion

50ml vegetable oil

1) egg

120ml boiling H20

For the icing:

50g butter at room temperature

50g icing sugar

Inch tablespoon matcha green tea powder.

1/2 tsp vanilla bean glue

50g Delicate cream

• pre heat the oven into 180C/160C admirer. Line a cup cake tin with either silicone or paper curry instances.

• Put the sugar, cocoa, Salt and espresso powder in a huge bowl and then mix carefully.

• Insert the vanilla, vanilla infusion, Vegetable egg and oil into the dry elements and also use a power mixer to beat till very well mixed. Gently pour into the boiling water lightly and conquer a very low rate until completely merged. Make use of a highspeed to be at to get a more minute in order to add atmosphere into the batter. The batter is far more liquid compared to the usual conventional curry mixture. Take religion, it is going to taste great!

• Spoon the batter equally between The cake instances. Just about every cake instance ought to really be no further than 3/4 entire. Bake in the oven for about 15 18 minutes, before mix pops once exploited. Remove from the oven and let it cool before icing.

• to Create the ice cream the Butter and icing sugar together until finally it truly is smooth and mild. Insert the matcha Vanilla and powder and stir fry. Finally put in the cream and beat till Simple. Pipe or disperse across the cakes.

SESAME CHICKEN SALAD-Sirtfood Recipes

304 calls • 3.5 of One's SIRT 5 per day

A yummy and unusual salad.

Serves 2 • All Set at 1 2 moments

1 tablespoon sesame seeds

1 pineapple, peeled, halved Length-ways, deseeded using a tsp plus chopped

100g infant spinach, approximately sliced

60g pack choir, finely painted

1/2 reddish onion, very finely chopped

Enormous number (20g) chopped, sliced

150g cooked poultry, shredded

For Your dressing:

1 tablespoon extra-virgin olive oil

1 teaspoon sesame oil

Juice of 1 lime

1 teaspoon clear honey

2 teaspoon soy sauce

Inch Toast the sesame seeds in a dry skillet for two minutes till lightly browned and aromatic. Move to a plate to cool.

Two In a little bowl, then combine the coconut oil, lavender oil, lime juice, soy, and honey sauce to create your dressing table.

3 Set the kale, carrot, pack choir, red onion and simmer into a huge bowl and then lightly blend with each other. Pour on the dressing and blend.

4 Spread the salad involving 2 plates and top with the chicken. Distribute within the sesame seeds right prior to serving.

Sir Food Mushroom Scramble Eggs-Sirtfood Recipes

Ingredients

2 tablespoon

Inch teaspoon ground garlic

Inch teaspoon mild curry powder

20g lettuce, approximately sliced

Inch teaspoon extra virgin Coconut Oil

1/2 Hen's eye peeled, thinly chopped

couple of mushrooms, finely chopped

5g parsley, finely chopped

*discretionary * Insert some seed mix for a topper and a few Rooster Sauce for taste

Guidelines

Blend the curry and garlic powder and then add just a small water till you've realized a mild glue.

Steam the lettuce 2-- three full moments.

Heat the oil into a skillet over a moderate heat and fry the chili and mushrooms to get 2-- three moments till they have begun to soften and brown.

Fragrant Chicken White Meat with Kale, Red Onion, along with Salsa-Sirtfood Recipes

Elements:

120g skinless, boneless chicken breast

2 tsp ground turmeric

Juice of 1/4 lemon

1 tablespoon extra-virgin olive oil

50g lettuce, sliced

20g red onion, chopped

1 teaspoon sliced fresh ginger

50g buckwheat

Guidelines:

To make the dinner, then eliminate the Attention From the tomato and then chop it rather finely, take good care to maintain up to this fluid as achievable. Mix using all the chili, capers, lemon, and carrot juice. You can put everything from a blender however that the result can be somewhat distinct.

Heat the oven to 220°C/petrol. Marinate the chicken white meat in 1 tsp of this garlic, the lemon juice and only a bit of oil. Leave 510 minutes.

Heat an ovenproof skillet before Sexy, you can put in the carrot and cook for one moment or so on both sides, until light gold, subsequently move for the oven (set on the baking dish in case a pan is not oven-proof) for 2 --10 seconds until cooked through. Remove from the oven, then cover with foil and leave to rest for five full minutes just before working out.

Meanwhile, cook kale at a Steamer for five full minutes. Stir the onions and the ginger at just a tiny oil until tender but not colored, you can add the carrot and simmer for one more moment.

Prepare the buckwheat in accordance with this Packet directions with all the rest teaspoon of garlic. Drink together with the poultry, broccoli and cauliflower.

Smoked Steak Omelet-Sirtfood Recipes

Try out this Fast and Effortless Sirtfood Dish packaged with goodness and flavor.

Serves:

Inch

Planning period:

5 -- 5 10 min

substances

two Moderate eggs

one hundred g Smoked salmon, sliced

1/2 tsp Capers

10 grams Rocket, sliced

inch teaspoon Parsley, sliced

inch teaspoon extra virgin coconut oil

Strategy

Combine the eggs to a bowl and then garnish well. Insert the salmon, capers, rocket and skillet.

Heat the coconut oil at a nontraditional skillet till extremely hot but not smoking cigarettes. Insert the egg mix and, with a spatula or fish slit, proceed the mix round the pan before it's even. Reduce heat and permit the omelet breathe. Twist the spatula round the edges and roll up or fold the omelet in half to function.

Green Tea Smoothie-Sirtfood Recipes

183 Energy

Inch of One's SIRT 5 per day

This super-healthy smoothie utilizes Matcha powder, and it is an extremely concentrated Japanese green tea. It might be located in Asian or tea outlets.

Serves 2 • Prepared in Three Minutes

2 ripe bananas

250 tsp milk

Two tsp matcha green tea powder

1/2 tsp vanilla bean glue (not infusion) or some little scratch of these seeds out of the vanilla pod

6 cubes

Two tsp honey

Simply mix each of the components Together at a blender and function in just two or two glasses.

CHAPTER FOUR
SESAME-SIRTFOOD RECIPES
SERVES Inch

Elements

20g miso

1 tablespoon mirin

Inch tablespoon extra-virgin Coconut Oil

200g skinless cod fillet

20g red onion, sliced

40g lettuce, sliced

Inch tsp clove, finely chopped

Inch bird's eye peeled, finely chopped

Inch teaspoon finely chopped fresh ginger

60g green legumes

50g lettuce, approximately sliced

Inch teaspoon unsalted seeds

5g tsp, roughly sliced

Inch tablespoon tamari

30g buckwheat

Inch teaspoon ground garlic

Guidelines

Mix that the miso, mirin, and One tsp of the petroleum. Rub all around the cod and leave to simmer for half an hour. Heat the oven to 220°C/petrol.

Bake the cod for 10 seconds.

Meanwhile, heat a Sizable skillet or combined using the oil. Insert the onion and then simmer to get a couple moments, add the garlic, celery, peppermint, peppermint, green lettuce, and beans. Toss and inhale till the kale is tender and cooked through. You might have to put in just a small water into the pan to assist the cooking procedure.

Prepare the buckwheat in accordance with this Packet directions with all the garlic for just 3 minutes.

Insert the sesame seeds, parsley and Tamari into the stir fry and function using the fish and greens.

Raspberry And black-currant Jelly-Sirtfood Recipes

Seventy-Six calories

Two of One's SIRT 5 per day

Getting a jelly beforehand is really a fantastic Means to ready the fresh fruit that it's about to consume first part of the daytime.

Serves 2 • All Set at a Quarter Hour + Setting timing

100g raspberries, Cleaned

2 renders gelatin

100g blackcurrants, Cleaned and Stalks eliminated

two tablespoon granulated sugar

300ml h2o

Inch Organize the desserts in 2 functioning dishes/glasses/molds. Set the gelatin leaves into a plate of water.

Two Put the blackcurrants in a little pan with all the glucose and also 100ml drinking water and then contribute to the boil. Simmer harshly for five full minutes then remove from the heating system. Leave stand for two weeks.

3 Squeeze excess water out of the gelatin leaves and then insert them into your batter. Squeeze until completely dissolved, then stir in the remainder of the drinking water. Pour the fluid in to the ready dishes and then refrigerate to place. The jellies ought to really be all set in roughly 34 minutes overnight.

Apple Pancakes using Black-currant Compote-Sirtfood Recipes

337 Energy

Inch 1/2 of you personally SIRT 5 per day

All these cakes are still decadent but Healthy. An excellent idle dawn cure.

Serves 4 • All Set at 20 minutes

75g porridge oats

125g plain yoghurt

1 teaspoon baking powder

Two tablespoon caster sugar

spoonful of salt

2 oranges, peeled, cored, and cut into little bits

300ml semi-skimmed milk

Two Egg-whites

Two teaspoon mild Essential Olive Oil

For Your compote:

120g blackcurrants, Cleaned and Stalks eliminated

two tablespoon caster sugar

3 tablespoons h2o

Inch To start creating the compote. Put the blackcurrants sugar and water in a little pan. Mention to a simmer and cook for 10 15 minutes.

Two Set the yogurt, milk, baking powder, then caster salt and sugar in a huge bowl and then mix nicely. Stir in the apple then whisk in the milk just a bit at some time before you are in possession of a clean mix. Whisk the egg whites into stiff peaks then fold in the pancake batter. Transfer the batter into some jug.

3 Warmth 1/2 teaspoon oil at a nontraditional skillet onto the medium-high heating and then pour into approximately 1 quarter of this batter. Cook both sides till gold brown. Eliminate and replicate to produce 4 pancakes.

4 Serve the sandwiches with all the black currant compote drizzled above.

SIRT Fresh fruit Salad- Sirtfood Recipes

172 Energy

3 of One's SIRT 5 per day

This fruit salad is packaged filled with The most optimal/optimally fresh fruit SIRTs.

Serves Inch • All Set at 10 moments

1/2 cup freshly produced Green-tea

1 teaspoon honey

Inch pear, coriander

Inch apple, cored and roughly sliced

10 red seedless grapes

10 blueberries

Inch Stir honey half of a cup of green tea extract. After simmer, add the juice half the orange peel. Leave cool.

Two Stir another 1 / 2 the orange and set into a bowl alongside all the chopped apple, blueberries and pears. Pour on the chilled tea and then leave to simmer for a couple moments before functioning.

SIRTFOOD BITES-SIRTFOOD RECIPES

Elements

120g walnuts

30g black chocolate (85 percent cocoa solids), broken to bits; or ginger nibs

250g Medjool dates, pitted

Inch tablespoon ginger powder

Inch tablespoon ground garlic

Inch tablespoon extra-virgin Coconut Oil

the cumin seeds of a single vanilla pod or One tsp vanilla infusion

Inch --two tablespoons Drinking Water

Guidelines

Set the chocolate and walnuts at a Food processor and process till you are in possession of a nice powder.

Insert the Rest of the components The mix and water till the mixture forms a chunk. Otherwise, you might or might well not need to bring the drinking water based upon the consequences of this mix -- that you really do not desire this to become overly tacky.

Together with your hands, shape the mix into bite-sized chunks and then refrigerate in an airtight container to get a minimum of 1 hour prior to ingesting them.

You can roll a Few of the chunks in A few more ginger or desiccated coconut to accomplish an alternative ending in the event you prefer.

They'll continue for one week Your refrigerator.

SIRT MUESLI-SIRTFOOD RECIPES

Elements:

20g buckwheat flakes

10g buckwheat puffs

15g coconut whites or desiccated Coconut

40g Medjool dates, pitted and Chopped

15g walnuts, sliced

10g cocoa nibs

100g strawberries, hulled and also Chopped

100g Ordinary Greek yogurt (or vegetarian Alternative (like soya or Coco Nut milk)

Guidelines:

Blend all the Aforementioned ingredients With each other, just including the oats and tomatoes prior to serving in the event you are which makes it at mass.

CHINESE-STYLE PORK WITH PAK CHOI-SIRTFOOD RECIPES

377 Energy AND two of One's SIRT 5 A-day

Serves 4

Elements

400g business tofu, cut into big cubes

1 tablespoon corn flour

1 tablespoon water

125ml chicken inventory

1 tablespoon rice

1 tablespoon tomato puree

1 teaspoon brown sugar

1 tablespoon soy sauce

1 tsp garlic, peeled and smashed

1 teaspoon (5cm) fresh ginger, peeled and grated 1 tablespoon rapeseed oil

100g shiitake mushrooms, sliced

1 teaspoon shallot, peeled and chopped

200g pack choir or choir amount, cut into thin pieces 400g pork mince (10 percent fat)

100g beansprouts

Large number (20g) parsley, sliced

Here is Just how:

Lay the kale out in kitchen newspaper, pay more toilet paper and place a side.

In a little bowl, then mix with the corn flour and water, then taking away all of lumps. Insert the chicken stock, rice, tomato puree, brown sugar, and soy sauce. Insert the smashed ginger and garlic and stir fry with them.

At a wok or large skillet, warm the oil into your top temperature. Insert the shiitake mushrooms stir-fry for two --three minutes before glossy and cooked. Get rid of the mushrooms in the pan using a slotted spoon and then place a side. Insert the carrot into the pan and then simmer until gold on either side. Take out using a slotted spoon and then place a side.

Insert the shallot and then pack choir into the wok, simmer for two weeks, adding the mince. Cook before the mince is cooked then put in the sauce, then cut back heat a notch and enable the sauce to bubble around the beef for one moment or 2. Insert the beansprouts, shiitake lettuce and mushrooms into the pan and heat. Take away from heat, stir the skillet and serve instantly.

Tuscan Bean Stew-Sirtfood Recipes

Elements

Inch tablespoon extra-virgin Coconut Oil

50g red onion, finely chopped

30g carrot, peeled and chopped

30g lettuce, trimmed and chopped

Inch garlic clove, finely chopped

1/2 Hen's eye peeled, finely chopped (optional)

Inch teaspoon herbs de Provence

200ml vegetable inventory

Inch x 400g tin chopped Italian berries

Inch teaspoon tomato purée

200g tinned Blended legumes

50g kale, approximately sliced

Inch tablespoon roughly chopped parsley

40g buckwheat

Technique

Set the oil in a medium saucepan Over a reduced --moderate heat and lightly fry the carrot, onion, garlic, celery, chili (if using) and herbaceous plants before onion is tender but not too colored.

Insert the stock, tomato and tomatoes purée and contribute to the boil. Insert the beans and simmer for half an hour.

Insert the carrot and cook another 510 minutes, till tender, and you can put in the skillet.

Meanwhile, prepare the buckwheat in line with the package directions, drain then serve using all the stew.

Salmon Shirt Tremendous Salad-Sirtfood Recipes

Helps Make Inch

Elements

50g rocket

50g chicory leaves

100g smoked salmon pieces (You Might Also Utilize legumes, cooked Chicken or tinned tuna)

80g avocado, peeled, stoned and chopped

40g celery, chopped

20g red onion, chopped

15g peppers, sliced

Inch tbs capers

Inch big Medjool Day, chopped and pitted

Inch tbs tsp Essential Olive Oil

Juice 1/4 lemon

10g tsp, sliced

10g lovage or celery leaves, sliced

Technique

Prepare the salad leaves onto a sizable plate. Blend all of the rest of the ingredients together and function on the surface of those leaves.

SIRTFOOD BITES

Serves 15 - 20 BITES

Elements:

1) cup (120g) walnuts

Inch oz (30g) black chocolate (Eighty-Five Percentage cocoa solids), broken to bits; or 1/4 cup ginger nibs

9 oz (250g) Medjool dates, pitted

1 tablespoon cocoa powder

1 tablespoon ground turmeric

1 tablespoon extra-virgin olive oil

The scraped seeds of inch carrot or one tsp vanilla infusion

1 or 2 tablespoon water

The Way to create:

Set the chocolate and walnuts at a Food processor and process till you are in possession of a nice powder.

Insert the Rest of the components The mix and water till the mixture forms a chunk. Otherwise, you might or might well not need to bring the drinking water based upon the consequences of this mix --that you really do not desire this to become overly tacky.

Together with your hands, shape the mix into bite-size chunks and then refrigerate in an airtight container for a minimum of 1 hour prior to ingesting them.

You can roll a Few of the chunks in A few more ginger dried coconuts to accomplish an alternative ending in the event you prefer. They'll endure for approximately 1 week on your own fridge.

SIRT Tremendous SALAD

Serves Inch

Elements:

1 3⁄4 oz (50g) arugula

1 3⁄4 oz (50g) endive leaves

3 1⁄2 oz (100g) smoked salmon Pieces

1⁄2 cup (80g) avocado, peeled, Stoned, also chopped

1⁄2 cup (50g) celery for example Leaves, chopped

1⁄8 cup (20g) red onion, sliced

1⁄8 cups (15g) walnuts, sliced

1 tablespoon capers

Inch big Medjool Day, pitted and Chopped

1 tablespoon extra-virgin olive oil

Juice of 1/4 lemon

1/4 cup (10g) parsley, sliced

The Way to create:

Set the salad leaves onto the plate at a big bowl.

Blend all of the ingredients that are remaining With each other and function on surface of these leaves.

MISO-MARINATED BAKED COD WITH Stir fried GREENS AND SESAME

Serves Inch

Elements:

3 1/2 tsp (20g) miso

1 tablespoon mirin

1 tablespoon extra-virgin olive oil

Inch x ray 7-ounce (200g) skinless cod fillet

1/8 cup (20g) red onion, sliced

3⁄8 cup (40g) celery, sliced

2 garlic cloves, finely chopped

Inch Thai chili, finely chopped

1 tsp thinly sliced fresh Ginger

3⁄8 cup (60g) green beans

3⁄4 cup (50g) kale, approximately sliced

1 tsp sesame seeds

2 tablespoon (5g) parsley, approximately Chopped

1 tablespoon tamari (or soy sauce, either If not preventing gluten)

1⁄4 cup (40g) buckwheat

1 tsp ground turmeric

The Way to create:

Mix that the miso, mirin, and One tsp of the petroleum. Rub throughout the cod and leave to simmer for half an hour. Heat the oven to 425oF (200oC).

Bake the cod for 10 seconds.

Meanwhile, heat a Sizable skillet or combined using the oil. Insert the onion and then simmer to get a couple moments, add the garlic, celery, ginger, coriander, green beans, as well as kale. Toss and inhale till the kale is tender and cooked through. You might have to put in just a tiny water into the pan to assist the cooking procedure.

Prepare the buckwheat in accordance with this Package directions as well as all the turmeric.

Insert the sesame seeds, parsley, and Tamari into the stir fry and function using all the buckwheat along with fish.

Fragrant Chicken WITH KALE AND RED ONIONS along with a TOMATO AND CHILI SALSA

Serves Inch

Elements:

1⁄4 pound (120g) skinless, boneless Chicken breast

2 tsp ground turmeric

Juice of 1/4 lemon

1 tablespoon extra-virgin olive oil

3/4 cup (50g) lettuce, sliced

1/8 cup (20g) red onion, sliced

1 tsp chopped fresh ginger

1/3 cup (50g) buckwheat

For Your SALSA

1 medium 1 (130g)

Inch Thai chili, finely chopped

1 tablespoon capers, finely chopped

2 tablespoon (5g) parsley, finely Chopped

Juice of 1/4 lemon

The Way to create:

To make the dinner, then eliminate the Attention From the tomato and then chop it rather finely, take good care to maintain up to this fluid as achievable. Mix using all the chili, capers, parsley, and lemon juice. You can put everything from a blender; however, the result can be really a bit distinct.

Heat the oven into 425°F (220°C). Marinate the egg into 1 tsp of this garlic, the lemon juice and only a bit of oil. Leave 5 to ten minutes.

Heat an ovenproof skillet before Sexy, you can put in the carrot and cook for one moment or so on both sides, until light gold, subsequently move for the oven (set on the baking dish in case a pan is not oven-proof) for 2 to ten minutes until cooked through. Remove from the oven, then cover with foil, and leave to sleep for five full minutes just before working out.

Meanwhile, cook kale at a Steamer for five full minutes. Stir the onions and the ginger at just a tiny oil until tender but not browned, you can add the carrot and simmer for one more moment.

Prepare the buckwheat in accordance with this Package instructions together with all the rest teaspoon of garlic. Drink together with the poultry vegetables, and also dinner.

ASIAN SHRIMP Stir Fry WITH BUCKWHEAT NOODLES

Serves Inch

Elements:

1/3 pound (150g) shelled raw jumbo shrimp, deveined

2 tsp tamari (You May utilize soy Sauce in the event that you aren't quitting gluten)

2 tsp extra virgin olive oil

3 oz (75g) soba (buckwheat Noodles)

2 garlic cloves, finely chopped

Inch Thai chili, finely chopped

1 tsp thinly sliced fresh Ginger

1/8 cup (20g) reddish onions, chopped

1/2 cup (45g) celery for example Leaves, trimmed and chopped, with leaves placed a side

1/2 cup (75g) green beans, sliced

3/4 cup (50g) kale, approximately sliced

½ cup (100ml) poultry inventory

The Way to create:

Heat a skillet on high heat, then prepare the fish into 1 tsp of this tamari and then one tsp of this oil to 2-3 minutes.

Transfer the fish to a plate. Wipe Out the pan having a paper towel as you are going to utilize it.

Prepare the noodles in boiling H20 for 5 to 8 minutes as directed on the offer. Drain and place a side.

Meanwhile, fry the garlic chili, Ginger, red onion, celery (however, maybe not exactly the leaves), green beans, and lettuce from the rest of the tamari and petroleum within medium-high warmth for two to three minutes. Insert the stock and bring to a boil, then simmer for one moment or 2, till the veggies have been cooked but still crispy.

Insert the beans, noodles, and celery Leaves into the pan, then return to a boil, then remove from heat and function.

STRAWBERRY BUCKWHEAT TABBOULEH

Serves Inch

Elements:

1⁄3 cup (50g) buckwheat

1 tablespoon ground turmeric

1⁄2 cup (80g) avocado

3⁄8 cup (65g) tomato

1⁄8 cup (20g) reddish onion

1⁄8 cup (25g) Medjool dates, pitted

1 tablespoon capers

3⁄4 cup (30g) skillet

2⁄3 cup (100g) strawberries, hulled

1 tablespoon extra-virgin olive oil

Juice of 1⁄2 lemon

Inch oz (30g) arugula

The Way to create:

Prepare the buckwheat together with all the garlic as stated by the program guidelines.

Drain and put aside to cool.

Finely chop the avocado, tomato, reddish Onion, dates, capers, and parsley and combine with all the trendy buckwheat.

Cut the berries and lightly Mix to the salad with all an oil along with lemon juice. Sit over a bed of arugula.

CHAPTER FIVE
SIRTFOOD GREEN JUICE
SIRTFOOD GREEN JUICE

Serves Inch

Elements:

2 big handfuls (roughly 2 1⁄2 oz or 75g) kale

a sizable amount (1 oz or 30g) arugula

a tiny number (approximately 1⁄4 oz or 5g) flat-leaf parsley

two to 3 large celery stalks (5 1⁄2 oz or 150g) (such as leaves

1/2 moderate green apple

1/2- to 1-inch (1 to 2 2.5 cm) piece of fresh ginger

juice of 1/2 lemon

1/2 amount teaspoon matcha powder

The Way to create:

Blend the greens (kale, arugula, and Parsley) collectively, then juice them. We detect that juicers really can change in their efficacy at leafy leafy veggies, and you also may possibly want to reduce the leftovers prior to continuing to other substances. The aim would be always to wind up with approximately two liquid ounce or near 1⁄4 cup (50ml) of juice in the greens.

Now juice the apple, celery and Ginger.

It's Possible for you to peel off the lemon and also place it Throughout the juicer too, however we still think it is a lot simpler to just squeeze the lemon hand in to the juice. With this phase, you ought to consume approximately 1) cup (250ml) of juice at total, most likely marginally more.

It is just Whenever the juice has been created and prepared to function that you simply put in the matcha. Put a little sum of the juice into a glass then put in the matcha and stir vigorously with a teaspoon or fork.

The Moment the matcha is excavated, insert The rest of the juice. Give it your final stir fry, after which your juice is about to beverage. Don't hesitate to top up using water that is plain according to preference.

The Sirtfood Juice

A Fantastic Way to Begin is using All the Sirtfood Juice -- thus we have thrown into the recipe for this to start out off you being a bonus further. The publication recommends drinking juices along with also adding inch meal to the initial 3 times, then two juices, then two meals to the subsequent 4 months. Sirtfood Green Juice (functions Inch)

Elements:

   2 big handfuls (75g) lettuce

   a Huge group (30g) rocket

   that an Exact Modest number (5g) flat-leaf parsley

   a Rather Small number (5g) lovage leaves (discretionary)

two --3 big stalks (150g) green lettuce, such as its own leaves

1/2 moderate green veggie

juice of 1/2 lemon

1/2 amount teaspoon matcha Green tea

Guidelines:

Blend the greens (ginseng, ginseng, Parsley and lovage (if applying) collectively, then juice them. We detect pitchers really can change within their efficacy at leafy veggies and you'll probably want to re-juice the leftovers prior to continuing to one additional substances. The aim will be to wind up getting approximately 50ml of juice out of the egg whites.

Now juice and apple. You Can peel off the lemon and then use it throughout the juicer also, however we still think it is a lot simpler to just squeeze the lemon hand in to juice. With this phase you must consume approximately 250ml of juice total, most likely marginally more. It is merely whenever the juice was created and prepared to function you simply add the matcha green tea extract.

Put a Small Quantity of the juice into a glass then put in the matcha and stir vigorously with a teaspoon or fork. We just utilize matcha from the initial two beverages of this afternoon since it comprises moderate levels of caffeine (the exact identical material being a standard cup of tea daily). For individuals not utilized for it, then it can maintain them alert in case drunk late. Once that the matcha is excavated include the rest of the juice.

Give it a final wake up, then your own Juice is about to beverage. Don't hesitate to top up using water that is plain according to preference.

Shirt Muesli (functions Inch)

If You Would like to Get This at mass or Prepare it the evening ahead, only merge the dry ingredients and save it at an airtight container. All you could have to do that the following day would be put in the berries and yogurt also it's really a good idea to really go.

Elements:

20g buckwheat tsp

10g buckwheat puffs

15g coconut tsp or desiccated coconut

40g Medjool dates, pitted and sliced

15g peppers, sliced

10g cocoa nibs

100g strawberries, hulled and sliced

100g Ordinary Greek yogurt (or vegetarian choice, for example soya or Coco Nut yoghurt)

Guidelines:

Blend all the above-Mentioned ingredients With each other (exit the berries and yoghurt in case maybe not functioning directly off).

Fragrant Chicken breast together with red and kale onions plus a tomato and chili salsa (functions inch)

Elements:

120g skinless, boneless Chicken

Two tsp ground garlic

juice of 1/4 lemon

Inch tablespoon extra-virgin Coconut Oil

50g lettuce, sliced

20g red onion, sliced

Inch teaspoon sliced fresh ginger

50g buckwheat

For Your supper

130g tomato (roughly 1))

Inch bird's eye chili, finely chopped

Inch tablespoon capers, finely chopped

5g tsp, finely chopped

Juice of 1/4 lemon

Guidelines:

To make the dinner, then eliminate the Attention From the tomato and then chop it rather finely, take good care to maintain up to this fluid as achievable. Mix using all the chili, capers, lemon, and carrot juice. You can put everything from a blender however that the result can be somewhat distinct.

Heat the oven to 220°C/petrol. Marinate the chicken white meat in 1 tsp of this garlic, the lemon juice and only a bit of oil. Leave 510 minutes. Heat a supplementary skillet until sizzling then put in the carrot and cook for one moment or so on both sides, until light gold, then move for the oven (set on the baking dish in case a pan is not oven-proof) for 2 --10 seconds until cooked through. Remove from the oven, then cover with foil and leave to rest for five full minutes just before working out.

Meanwhile, cook kale at a Steamer for five full minutes. Stir the onions and the ginger at just a tiny oil until tender but not colored, you can add the carrot and simmer for one more minute. Cook that the buckwheat in line with the package guidelines with all the rest teaspoon of garlic. Drink together with the poultry, broccoli and cauliflower.

Sirtfood Snacks (leaves 1520 snacks)

Elements:

120g walnuts

30g black chocolate (85 percent cocoa solids), broken to bits; or ginger nibs

250g Medjool dates, pitted

Inch tablespoon ginger powder

Inch tablespoon ground garlic

Inch tablespoon extra-virgin Coconut Oil

the cumin seeds of 1 teaspoon carrot or One tsp vanilla infusion

Inch --two tablespoons Drinking Water

Guidelines:

Set the chocolate and walnuts at a Food processor and process till you are in possession of a nice powder.

Insert the rest of the ingredients besides the drinking water and mix till the mixture forms a chunk. Otherwise, you might or might well not need to bring the drinking water based upon the consequences of this mix -- that you really do not desire this to become overly tacky.

Together with your hands, shape the mix into bite-sized chunks and then refrigerate in an airtight container for a minimum of 1 hour prior to ingesting them. You'll roll a few of the chunks in a few more ginger or desiccated coconut to accomplish an alternative finish in the event you would like. They'll endure for approximately 1 week on your own fridge.

Asian King prawn stir fry with buckwheat noodles (functions inch)

Elements:

150g shelled raw king prawns, deveined

Two tsp tamari (You May utilize soy sauce if You Aren't preventing gluten)

Two teaspoon extra virgin coconut oil

75g soba (buckwheat noodles)

Inch tsp clove, finely chopped

Inch bird's eye chili, finely chopped

Inch teaspoon finely chopped fresh ginger

20g red onions, chopped

40g celery, trimmed and chopped

75g green beans, sliced

50g kale, approximately sliced

100ml poultry inventory

5g lovage or lettuce leaves

Guidelines:

Heat a skillet on a high warmth, then prepare the prawns into 1 tsp of this tamari and then one tsp of this oil 2--three full minutes. Transfer the prawns into some plate. Wipe out the pan using kitchen paper, even since you are definitely going to utilize it.

Prepare the noodles in boiling H2o for 5minutes as directed on the package. Drain and place a side.

Meanwhile, fry the garlic, peppermint and ginger, red celery, onion, legumes, and lettuce at the rest of the oil over a moderate --higher temperature for two --three full moments. Insert the stock and bring to the boil, then simmer for one moment or 2, before veggies have been cooked but still crispy.

Insert the prawns, noodles along with Lovage/celery leaves into the pan, then return to the boil then remove from heat and function.

Strawberry buckwheat tabbouleh

Elements:

50g buckwheat

Inch tablespoon ground turmeric

80g avocado

65g tomato

20g red berry

25g Medjool dates, pitted

Inch tablespoon capers

30g parsley

100g strawberries, hulled

Inch tablespoon extra-virgin Coconut Oil

juice of 1/2 lemon

30g rocket

Guidelines:

Prepare the buckwheat together with all the garlic as stated by the package directions. Drain and continue to a side to trendy.

Finely chop the avocado, tomato, reddish Onion, dates, capers and mix with all the trendy buckwheat. Cut the berries and lightly mix in the salad with all an oil and lemon juice. Sit over a bed.

Sirtfood Diet programs

We have chosen a few of our Favored recipes out of the publication to secure you started out.

Elements:

20g buckwheat flakes

10g buckwheat puffs

15g coconut whites or desiccated Coconut

40g Medjool dates, pitted and Chopped

15g walnuts, sliced

10g cocoa nibs

100g strawberries, hulled and also Chopped

100g Ordinary Greek yogurt (or vegetarian Alternative (like soya or Coco Nut milk)

Guidelines:

Blend all the Aforementioned ingredients With each other, just including the oats and berries prior to working out in case your earning it mass.

Steak: Tuscan Bean Stew

Elements:

1 tablespoon extra-virgin olive oil

50g red onion, finely chopped

30g carrot, peeled and finely Chopped

30g lettuce, trimmed and finely Chopped

1 garlic clove, finely chopped

1/2 Hen's eye chili, finely chopped (optional)

Inch teaspoon herbs de Provence

200ml vegetable inventory

1 x 400g tin chopped Italian Berries

1 teaspoon tomato purée

200g tinned Blended legumes

50g kale, approximately sliced

1 tablespoon roughly chopped parsley

40g buckwheat

Instructions:

Set the oil in a medium saucepan Over a reduced --moderate heat and lightly stir the carrot, onion, garlic, celery, chili, when using herbs and herbaceous plants, before onion is tender but not colored.

Insert the berries and tomatoes Purée and contribute to the boil.

Insert the beans and simmer for 30 Moments.

Insert the carrot and cook for a Different 5-- 5 10 minutes, till tender, and you can put in the skillet.

Meanwhile, Prepare the buckwheat as stated by the packet directions, drain then serve using all the stew.

Evening Meal: Fragrant Chicken breast together with Kale, Red Onion, along with Salsa

Elements:

120g skinless, boneless chicken breast

2 tsp ground turmeric

Juice of 1/4 lemon

1 tablespoon extra-virgin olive oil

50g lettuce, sliced

20g red onion, chopped

1 teaspoon sliced fresh ginger

50g buckwheat

Instructions:

To make the dinner, then eliminate the Attention From the tomato and then chop it rather finely, take good care to maintain up to this fluid as achievable. Mix using all the chili, capers, lemon, and carrot juice. You can put everything from a blender however that the result can be somewhat distinct.

Heat the oven to 220°C/petrol. Marinate the chicken white meat in 1 tsp of this garlic, the lemon juice and only a bit of oil. Leave 510 minutes.

Heat an ovenproof skillet before Sexy, you can put in the carrot and cook for one moment or so on both sides, until light gold, subsequently move for the oven (set on the baking dish in case a pan is not oven-proof) for 2 --10 seconds until cooked through. Remove from the oven, then cover with foil and leave to rest for five full minutes just before working out.

Meanwhile, cook kale at a Steamer for five full minutes. Stir the onions and the ginger at just a tiny oil until tender but not colored, you can add the carrot and simmer for one more moment.

Prepare the buckwheat in accordance with this Packet direction with all the rest teaspoon of garlic. Serve along Side The poultry vegetables and salsa.

CHAPTER SIX
RECIPES
THE SIRTFOOD DIET GREEN JUICE

Course: Drink, Juice

Cuisine: British

Prep Time5 minutes

All out Time5 minutes

Servings1

Fixings

- 75 g kale

- 30 g rocket

- 5 g parsley

- 2 celery sticks

- ½ green apple

- 1 cm ginger

- Juice of ½ lemon

- ½ teaspoon matcha green tea

Guidelines

1.   Juice all the fixings separated from the lemon and the matcha green tea.

2.   Squeeze the lemon juice into the green squeeze by hand.

3.   Pour a limited quantity of green juice into a glass and mix in the matcha. Include the remainder of the green juice into the glass and mix once more.

4.   Drink straight away or put something aside for some other time.

MISO-MARINATED BAKED COD WITH STIR-FRIED GREENS AND SESAME

SERVES 1

Fixings:

- 3 ½ teaspoons (20g) miso

- 1 tablespoon mirin

- 1 tablespoon additional virgin olive oil

- 1 x 7-ounce (200g) skinless cod filet

- ⅛ cup (20g) red onion, cut

- ⅜ cup (40g) celery, cut

- 2 garlic cloves, finely hacked

- 1 Thai stew, finely cleaved

- 1 teaspoon finely hacked new ginger

- ⅜ cup (60g) green beans

- ¾ cup (50g) kale, generally cleaved

- 1 teaspoon sesame seeds

- 2 tablespoons (5g) parsley, generally cleaved

- 1 tablespoon tamari (or soy sauce, if not evading gluten)

- ¼ cup (40g) buckwheat

- 1 teaspoon ground turmeric

Method:

- Blend the miso, mirin, and 1 teaspoon of the oil. Rub everywhere throughout the cod and leave to marinate for 30 minutes. Warmth the stove to 4250F (2200C).

- Prepare the cod for 10 minutes.

- In the interim, heat a huge skillet or wok with the rest of the oil. Include the onion and sautéed food for a couple of moments, at that point include the celery, garlic, stew, ginger, green beans, and kale. Hurl and fry until the kale is delicate and cooked through. You may need to add a little water to the dish to help the cooking procedure.

- Cook the buckwheat as indicated by the bundle directions along with the turmeric.

- Include the sesame seeds, parsley, and tamari to the sautéed food and present with the buckwheat and fish.

SIRTFOOD BITES

SERVES 15 - 20 BITES

Fixings:

- 1 cup (120g) pecans

- 1 ounce (30g) dim chocolate (85 percent cocoa solids), broken into pieces; or ¼ cup cocoa nibs

- 9 ounces (250g) Medjool dates, pitted

- 1 tablespoon cocoa powder

- 1 tablespoon ground turmeric

- 1 tablespoon additional virgin olive oil

- the scratched seeds of 1 vanilla unit or 1 teaspoon vanilla concentrate

- 1 to 2 tablespoons water

Instruction:

- Spot the pecans and chocolate in a food processor and procedure until you have a fine powder.

- Include the various fixings aside from the water and mix until the blend shapes a ball. You could possibly need to include the water depending the consistency of the blend—you don't need it to be excessively clingy.

- Utilizing your hands, structure the blend into reduced down balls and refrigerate in a sealed shut holder for in any event 1 hour before eating them.

- You could move a portion of the balls in some more cocoa or dried coconut to accomplish an alternate completion on the off chance that you like. They will keep for as long as multi week in your ice chest.

SIRT SUPER SALAD

SERVES 1

Fixings:

- 1 3/4 ounces (50g) arugula

- 1 3/4 ounces (50g) endive leaves

- 3 ½ ounces (100g) smoked salmon cuts

- ½ cup (80g) avocado, stripped, stoned, and cut

- ½ cup (50g) celery including leaves, cut

- ⅛ cup (20g) red onion, cut

- ⅛ cups (15g) pecans, hacked

- 1 tablespoon tricks

- 1 huge Medjool date, hollowed and hacked

- 1 tablespoon additional virgin olive oil

- juice of ¼ lemon

- ¼ cup (10g) parsley, slashed

Instruction:

Spot the serving of mixed greens leaves on a plate or in a huge bowl.

Combine all the rest of the fixings and serve on the leaves.

SWEET-SMELLING CHICKEN BREAST WITH KALE AND RED ONIONS AND A TOMATO AND CHILI SALSA

SERVES 1

Fixings:

- ¼ pound (120g) skinless, boneless chicken bosom

- 2 teaspoons ground turmeric

- juice of ¼ lemon

- 1 tablespoon additional virgin olive oil

- 3⁄4 cup (50g) kale, slashed

- 1⁄8 cup (20g) red onion, cut

- 1 teaspoon slashed new ginger

- 1⁄3 cup (50g) buckwheat

FOR THE SALSA

- 1 medium tomato (130g)

- 1 Thai bean stew, finely cleaved

- 1 tablespoon escapades, finely cleaved

- 2 tablespoons (5g) parsley, finely slashed

- juice of 1⁄4 lemon

Instruction:

- To make the salsa, expel the eye from the tomato and slash it finely, taking consideration to keep however much of the fluid as could be expected. Blend in with the bean stew, escapades, parsley, and lemon juice. You could place everything in a blender, however the final product is somewhat extraordinary.

- Warmth the broiler to 425°F (220°C). Marinate the chicken bosom in 1 teaspoon of the turmeric, the lemon juice, and a little oil. Leave for 5 to 10 minutes.

- Warmth an ovenproof griddle until hot, at that point include the marinated chicken and cook for a moment or so on each side, until pale brilliant, at that point move to the stove (place on a heating plate if your skillet isn't ovenproof) for 8 to 10 minutes or until cooked through. Expel from the stove, spread with foil, and leave to rest for 5 minutes before serving.

- In the meantime, cook the kale in a liner for 5 minutes. Fry the red onions and the ginger in a little oil, until delicate yet not sautéed, at that point include the cooked kale and fry for one more moment.

- Cook the buckwheat as per the bundle guidelines with the rest of the teaspoon of turmeric. Serve close by the chicken, vegetables, and salsa.

ASIAN SHRIMP STIR-FRY WITH BUCKWHEAT NOODLES

SERVES 1

Fixings:

- 1/3 pound (150g) shelled crude large shrimp, deveined

- 2 teaspoons tamari (you can utilize soy sauce in the event that you are not staying away from gluten)

- 2 teaspoons additional virgin olive oil

- 3 ounces (75g) soba (buckwheat noodles)

- 2 garlic cloves, finely slashed

- 1 Thai bean stew, finely slashed

- 1 teaspoon finely slashed new ginger

- 1/8 cup (20g) red onions, cut

- 1/2 cup (45g) celery including leaves, cut and cut, with leaves put in a safe spot

- ½ cup (75g) green beans, slashed

- ¾ cup (50g) kale, generally slashed

- ½ cup (100ml) chicken stock

Instruction:

- Warmth a griddle over high warmth, at that point cook the shrimp in 1 teaspoon of the tamari and 1 teaspoon of the oil for 2 to 3 minutes.

- Move the shrimp to a plate. Wipe the work out with a paper towel, as you're going to utilize it once more.

- Cook the noodles in bubbling water for 5 to 8 minutes or as coordinated on the bundle. Channel and put in a safe spot.

- Then, fry the garlic, stew, ginger, red onion, celery (however not the leaves), green beans, and kale in the remaining tamari and oil over medium-high warmth for 2 to 3 minutes. Add the stock and heat to the point of boiling, at that point stew for a moment or two, until the vegetables are cooked yet at the same time crunchy.

- Include the shrimp, noodles, and celery leaves to the container, heat back to the point of boiling, at that point expel from the warmth and serve.

STRAWBERRY BUCKWHEAT TABBOULEH

SERVES 1

Fixings:

- ⅓ cup (50g) buckwheat

- 1 tablespoon ground turmeric

- ½ cup (80g) avocado

- 3⁄8 cup (65g) tomato

- 1⁄8 cup (20g) red onion

- 1⁄8 cup (25g) Medjool dates, pitted

- 1 tablespoon escapades

- 3⁄4 cup (30g) parsley

- 2⁄3 cup (100g) strawberries, hulled

- 1 tablespoon additional virgin olive oil

- juice of ½ lemon

- 1 ounce (30g) arugula

Instruction:

- Cook the buckwheat with the turmeric as per the bundle directions.

- Channel and put aside to cool.

- Finely hack the avocado, tomato, red onion, dates, tricks, and parsley and blend in with the cool buckwheat.

- Cut the strawberries and tenderly blend into the serving of mixed greens with the oil and lemon juice. Serve on a bed of arugula.

SIRTFOOD GREEN JUICE

SERVES 1

Fixings:

- 2 huge bunches (around 2 ½ ounces or 75g) kale

- a huge bunch (1 ounce or 30g) arugula

- a little bunch (about ¼ ounce or 5g) level leaf parsley

- 2 to 3 huge celery stems (5 ½ ounces or 150g), including leaves

- 1/2 medium green apple

- 1/2-to 1-inch (1 to 2.5 cm) bit of new ginger

- juice of 1/2 lemon

- 1/2 level teaspoon matcha powder

Instruction:

- Blend the greens (kale, arugula, and parsley) together, at that point juice them. We find that juicers can truly vary in their proficiency at squeezing verdant vegetables, and you may need to reduce the leftovers before proceeding onward to different fixings. The objective is to wind up with around 2 liquid ounces or near ¼ cup (50ml) of juice from the greens.

- Presently squeeze the celery, apple, and ginger.

- You can strip the lemon and put it through the juicer also, however we think that it's a lot simpler to just crush the lemon by hand into the juice. By this stage, you ought to have around 1 cup (250ml) of juice altogether, maybe somewhat more.

- It is just when the juice is made and prepared to serve that you include the matcha. Pour a limited quantity of the juice into a glass, at that point include the matcha and mix enthusiastically with a fork or teaspoon.

- Once the matcha is broken down, include the rest of the juice. Give it a last mix, at that point your juice is prepared to drink. Don't hesitate to top up with plain water, as indicated by taste.

MIXED OMELET TOAST TOPPER

Fixings

- 2 eggs

- 1 tbsp crème fraiche

- 25g cheddar, ground

- little pack chive, clipped

- 1 spring onion, cut

- 1 tsp oil

- 3-4 cherry tomatoes, split

- 2 cups dried up bread, toasted

Strategy

- Beat together eggs, crème fraiche, cheddar, and chives with a touch of flavoring. Warmth oil in a skillet, at that point relax spring onion for a couple of minutes. Include tomatoes and warm through, at that point pour in egg blend. Cook over a low warmth, mixing, until eggs are simply set. Heap over toast.

TURMERIC CHICKEN and KALE SALAD WITH HONEY LIME DRESSING-SIRTFOOD RECIPES

Notes: If getting ready early, dress the plate of mixed greens 10 minutes before serving. Chicken can be supplanted with hamburger mince, cleaved prawns or fish. Veggie lovers could utilize slashed mushrooms or cooked quinoa.

Serves: 2

Fixings

For the chicken

* 1 teaspoon ghee or 1 tbsp coconut oil

* ½ medium earthy colored onion, diced

* 250-300 g/9 oz. chicken mince or diced up chicken thighs

* 1 enormous garlic clove, finely diced

* 1 teaspoon turmeric powder

* 1teaspoon lime pizzazz

* juice of ½ lime

* ½ teaspoon salt + pepper

For the serving of mixed greens

* 6 broccolini stalks or 2 cups of broccoli florets

* 2 tablespoons pumpkin seeds (pepitas)

* 3 enormous kale leaves, stems evacuated and cleaved

* ½ avocado, cut

* bunch of new coriander leaves, cleaved

* bunch of new parsley leaves, cleaved

For the dressing

* 3 tablespoons lime juice

* 1 little garlic clove, finely diced or ground

* 3 tablespoons extra-virgin olive oil (I utilized 1 tablespoon avocado oil and * 2 tablespoons EVO)

*1 teaspoon crude nectar

* ½ teaspoon wholegrain or Dijon mustard

* ½ teaspoon ocean salt and pepper

Directions

1. Warmth the ghee or coconut oil in a little skillet over medium-high warmth. Include the onion and sauté medium warmth for 4-5 minutes, until brilliant. Include the chicken mince and garlic and mix for 2-3 minutes over medium-high warmth, breaking it separated.

2. Include the turmeric, lime get-up-and-go, lime squeeze, salt and pepper and cook, blending much of the time, for a further 3-4 minutes. Put the cooked mince in a safe spot.

3. While the chicken is cooking, carry a little pot of water to bubble. Include the broccolini and cook for 2 minutes. Wash under virus water and cut into 3-4 pieces each.

4. Add the pumpkin seeds to the skillet from the chicken and toast over medium warmth for 2 minutes, mixing oftentimes to forestall consuming. Season with somewhat salt. Put in a safe spot. Crude pumpkin seeds are additionally fine to utilize.

5. Spot hacked kale in a plate of mixed greens amaze and pour the dressing. Utilizing your hands, hurl and back rub the kale with the dressing. This will mellow the kale, sort of like what citrus juice does to fish or hamburger carpaccio – it 'cooks' it somewhat.

6. At long last hurl through the cooked chicken, broccolini, new herbs, pumpkin seeds and avocado cuts.

BUCKWHEAT NOODLES WITH CHICKEN KALE and MISO DRESSING-SIRTFOOD RECIPES

Serves: 2

Fixings

For the noodles

* 2-3 bunches of kale leaves (expelled from the stem and generally cut)

* 150 g/5 oz buckwheat noodles (100% buckwheat, no wheat)

* 3-4 shiitake mushrooms, cut

* 1 teaspoon coconut oil or ghee

* 1 earthy colored onion, finely diced

* 1 medium unfenced chicken bosom, cut or diced

* 1 long red bean stew, meagerly cut (seeds in or out contingent upon how hot you like it)

* 2 enormous garlic cloves, finely diced

* 2-3 tablespoons Tamari sauce (without gluten soy sauce)

For the miso dressing

* 1½ tablespoon new natural miso

* 1 tablespoon Tamari sauce

* 1 tablespoon extra-virgin olive oil

* 1 tablespoon lemon or lime juice

* 1 teaspoon sesame oil (discretionary)

Guidelines

1. Carry a medium pot of water to bubble. Include the kale and cook for 1 moment, until somewhat withered. Expel and put in a safe spot however hold the water and take it back to the bubble. Include the soba noodles and cook as per the bundle guidelines (generally around 5 minutes). Wash under virus water and put in a safe spot.

2. Meanwhile, sear the shiitake mushrooms in a little ghee or coconut oil (about a teaspoon) for 2-3 minutes, until daintily caramelized on each side. Sprinkle with ocean salt and put in a safe spot.

3. In a similar skillet, heat more coconut oil or ghee over medium-high warmth. Sauté onion and bean stew for 2-3 minutes and afterward include the chicken pieces. Cook 5 minutes over medium warmth, blending a few times, at that point include the garlic, tamari sauce and a little sprinkle of water. Cook for a further 2-3 minutes, blending every now and again until chicken is cooked through.

4. At long last, include the kale and soba noodles and hurl through the chicken to heat up.

5.Mix the miso dressing and sprinkle over the noodles directly toward the finish of cooking, along these lines you will keep every one of those advantageous probiotics in the miso alive and dynamic.

ASIAN KING PRAWN STIR-FRY WITH BUCKWHEAT NOODLES

Serves 1

Fixings:

- 150g shelled crude lord prawns, deveined

- 2 tsp tamari (you can utilize soy sauce in the event that you are not maintaining a strategic distance from gluten)

- 2 tsp additional virgin olive oil

- 75g soba (buckwheat noodles)

- 1 garlic clove, finely hacked

- 1 10,000-foot bean stew, finely cleaved

- 1 tsp finely hacked new ginger

- 20g red onions, cut

- 40g celery, cut and cut

- 75g green beans, hacked

- 50g kale, generally hacked

- 100ml chicken stock

- 5g lavage or celery leaves

Directions:

- Warmth a skillet over a high warmth, at that point cook the prawns in 1 teaspoon of the tamari and 1 teaspoon of the oil for 2–3 minutes. Move the prawns to a plate. Wipe the work out with kitchen paper, as you're going to utilize it once more.

- Cook the noodles in bubbling water for 5–8 minutes or as coordinated on the parcel. Channel and put in a safe spot.

- In the meantime, fry the garlic, stew and ginger, red onion, celery, beans and kale in the rest of the oil over a medium–high warmth for 2–3 minutes. Add the stock and bring to the bubble, at that point stew for a moment or two, until the vegetables are cooked yet at the same time crunchy.

- Include the prawns, noodles and lovage/celery leaves to the dish, take back to the bubble at that point expel from the warmth and serve.

HEATED SALMON SALAD WITH CREAMY MINT DRESSING

Heating the salmon in the broiler makes this serving of mixed greens so straightforward.

- 1 salmon filet (130g)

- 40g blended plate of mixed greens leaves

- 40g youthful spinach leaves

- 2 radishes, cut and daintily cut

- 5cm piece (50g) cucumber, cut into lumps

- 2 spring onions, cut and cut

- 1 little bunch (10g) parsley, generally hacked

- For the dressing:

- 1 tsp low-fat mayonnaise

- 1 tbsp characteristic yogurt

- 1 tbsp rice vinegar

- 2 leaves mint, finely hacked

- Salt and newly ground dark pepper

Instruction:

1 Preheat the stove to 200°C (180°C fan/Gas 6).

2 Place the salmon filet on a preparing plate and heat for 16–18 minutes until simply cooked through. Expel from the broiler and put in a safe spot. The salmon is similarly decent hot or cold in the plate of mixed greens. On the off chance that your salmon has skin, basically cook skin side down and expel the salmon from the skin utilizing a fish cut in the wake of cooking. It should slide off effectively when cooked.

3 In a little bowl, combine the mayonnaise, yogurt, rice wine vinegar, mint leaves and salt and pepper together and leave to represent in any event 5 minutes to permit the flavors to create.

4 Arrange the plate of mixed greens leaves and spinach on a serving plate and top with the radishes, cucumber, spring onions and parsley. Drop the cooked salmon onto the serving of mixed greens and shower the dressing over.

CHOC CHIP GRANOLA-SIRTFOOD RECIPES

Chocolate at breakfast! Make certain to present with some green tea to give you a lot of SIRTs. The rice malt syrup can be subbed with maple syrup on the off chance that you like.

- 200g kind sized oats

- 50g walnuts, generally slashed

- 3 tbsp light olive oil

- 20g margarine

- 1 tbsp dim earthy colored sugar

- 2 tbsp rice malt syrup

- 60g great quality (70%)

- dim chocolate chips

Instruction:

1 Preheat the broiler to 160°C (140°C fan/Gas 3). Line a huge heating plate with a silicone sheet or preparing material.

2 Mix the oats and walnuts together in an enormous bowl. In a little non-stick container, delicately heat the olive oil, margarine, earthy colored sugar and rice malt syrup until the spread has softened and the sugar and syrup have disintegrated. Try not to permit to bubble. Pour the syrup over the oats and mix altogether until the oats are completely secured.

3 Distribute the granola over the heating plate, spreading directly into the corners. Leave clusters of blend with dispersing as opposed to an even spread. Prepare in the broiler for 20 minutes until just tinged brilliant earthy colored at the edges. Expel from the broiler and leave to cool on the plate totally.

4 When cool, separate any greater irregularities on the plate with your fingers and afterward blend in the chocolate chips. Scoop or empty the granola into an impenetrable tub or container. The granola will save for in any event fourteen days.

FRAGRANT ASIAN HOTPOT-SIRTFOOD RECIPES

- 1 tsp tomato purée

- 1-star anise, squashed (or 1/4 tsp ground anise)

- Little bunch (10g) parsley, follows finely cleaved

- Little bunch (1Og) coriander, follows finely cleaved

- Juice of 1/2 lime

- 500ml chicken stock, new or made with 1 3D square

- 1/2 carrot, stripped and cut into matchsticks

- 50g broccoli, cut into little florets

- 50g beansprouts

- 100g crude tiger prawns

- 100g firm tofu, hacked

- 50g rice noodles, cooked by bundle guidelines

- 50g cooked water chestnuts, depleted

- 20g sushi ginger, slashed

- 1 tbsp great quality miso glue

Instruction:
- Spot the tomato purée, star anise, parsley stalks, coriander stalks, lime juice and chicken stock in a huge skillet and bring to a stew for 10 minutes.
- Include the carrot, broccoli, prawns, tofu, noodles and water chestnuts and stew delicately until the prawns are cooked through. Expel from the warmth and mix in the sushi ginger and miso glue.
- Serve sprinkled with the parsley and coriander leaves.

LAMB, BUTTERNUT SQUASH AND DATE TAGINE

Mind boggling warming Moroccan flavors make this solid tagine ideal for crisp harvest time and winter nights. Present with buckwheat for an additional wellbeing kick!

Serves: 4

Fixings

- 2 tablespoons olive oil

- 1 red onion, cut

- 2cm ginger, ground

- 3 garlic cloves, ground or squashed

- 1 teaspoon stew chips (or to taste)

- 2 teaspoons cumin seeds

- 1 cinnamon stick

- 2 teaspoons ground turmeric

- 800g sheep neck filet, cut into 2cm pieces

- ½ teaspoon salt

- 100g Medrol dates, hollowed and hacked

- 400g tin hacked tomatoes, in addition to a large portion of a container of water

- 500g butternut squash, hacked into 1cm 3D squares

- 400g tin chickpeas, depleted

- 2 tablespoons new coriander (in addition to extra for embellish)

- Buckwheat, couscous, flatbreads or rice to serve

Technique

1. Preheat your broiler to 140C.

2. Drizzle around 2 tablespoons of olive oil into an enormous ovenproof pot or cast iron goulash dish. Include the cut onion and cook on a delicate warmth, with the cover on, for around 5 minutes, until the onions are mollified yet not earthy colored.

3. Add the ground garlic and ginger, bean stew, cumin, cinnamon and turmeric. Mix well and cook for 1 progressively minute with the top off. Include a sprinkle of water on the off chance that it gets excessively dry.

4. Next include the sheep pieces. Mix well to cover the meat in the onions and flavors and afterward include the salt, slashed dates and tomatoes, in addition to about a large portion of a jar of water (100-200ml).

5. Bring the tagine to the bubble and afterward put the cover on and put in your preheated stove for 1 hour and 15 minutes.

6. Thirty minutes before the finish of the cooking time, include the cleaved butternut squash and depleted chickpeas. Mix everything together, set the top back on and come back to the stove for the last 30 minutes of cooking.

7. When the tagine is prepared, expel from the broiler and mix through the hacked coriander. Present with buckwheat, couscous, flatbreads or basmati rice.

Notes

In the event that you don't possess an ovenproof pot or cast iron goulash dish, basically cook the tagine in a standard pot up until it needs to go in the broiler and afterward move the tagine into an ordinary lidded meal dish before putting in the stove. Extra an additional 5 minutes cooking time to consider the way that the goulash dish will require additional opportunity to warm up.

PRAWN ARRABBIATA-SIRTFOOD RECIPES

Fixings

- 125-150 g Raw or cooked prawns (Ideally ruler prawns)

- 65 g Buckwheat pasta

- 1 tbsp Extra virgin olive oil

- For arrabbiata sauce

- 40 g Red onion, finely cleaved

- 1 Garlic clove, finely cleaved

- 30 g Celery, finely cleaved

- 1 Bird's eye bean stew, finely cleaved

- 1 tsp Dried blended herbs

- 1 tsp Extra virgin olive oil

- 2 tbsp White wine (discretionary)

- 400 g Tinned cleaved tomatoes

- 1 tbsp Chopped parsley

Strategy

1. Fry the onion, garlic, celery and bean stew and dried herbs in the oil over a medium–low warmth for 1–2 minutes. Turn the warmth up to medium, include the wine and cook for 1 moment. Include the tomatoes and leave the sauce to stew over a medium–low warmth for 20–30 minutes, until it has a pleasant rich consistency. On the off chance that you feel the sauce is getting too thick essentially include a little water.

2. While the sauce is cooking carry a skillet of water to the bubble and cook the pasta as per the bundle directions. At the point when cooked exactly as you would prefer, channel, hurl with the olive oil and keep in the container until required.

3. On the off chance that you are utilizing crude prawns add them to the sauce and cook for a further 3–4 minutes, until they have turned pink and dark, include the parsley and serve. On the off chance that you are utilizing cooked prawns include them with the parsley, carry the sauce to the bubble and serve.

4. Add the cooked pasta to the sauce, blend completely yet tenderly and serve.

TURMERIC BAKED SALMON-SIRTFOOD RECIPES

Fixings

- 125-150 g Skinned Salmon
- 1 tsp Extra virgin olive oil
- 1 tsp Ground turmeric
- 1/4 Juice of a lemon
- For the zesty celery
- 1 tsp Extra virgin olive oil
- 40 g Red onion, finely cleaved
- 60 g Tinned green lentils
- 1 Garlic clove, finely cleaved
- 1 cm Fresh ginger, finely cleaved
- 1 Bird's eye bean stew, finely cleaved
- 150 g Celery, cut into 2cm lengths
- 1 tsp Mild curry powder
- 130 g Tomato, cut into 8 wedges
- 100 ml Chicken or vegetable stock
- 1 tbsp Chopped parsley

Strategy

- Heat the stove to 200C/gas mark 6.

- Start with the zesty celery. Warmth a skillet over a medium–low warmth, include the olive oil, at that point the onion, garlic, ginger, bean stew and celery. Fry tenderly for 2–3 minutes or until mollified however not shaded, at that point include the curry powder and cook for a further moment.

- Add the tomatoes then the stock and lentils and stew tenderly for 10 minutes. You might need to increment or decline the cooking time contingent upon how crunchy you like your celery.

- Meanwhile, blend the turmeric, oil and lemon squeeze and rub over the salmon. # Place on a heating plate and cook for 8–10 minutes.

- To complete, mix the parsley through the celery and present with the salmon.

CORONATION CHICKEN SALAD

Fixings

- 75 g Natural yogurt

- Juice of 1/4 of a lemon

- 1 tsp Coriander, hacked

- 1 tsp Ground turmeric

- 1/2 tsp Mild curry powder

- 100 g Cooked chicken bosom, cut into scaled down pieces

- 6 Walnut parts, finely hacked

- 1 Medjool date, finely hacked

- 20 g Red onion, diced

- 1 Bird's eye stew

- 40 g Rocket, to serve

Strategy

- Blend the yogurt, lemon juice, coriander and flavors together in a bowl. Include all the rest of the fixings and serve on a bed of the rocket.

PREPARED POTATOES WITH SPICY CHICKPEA STEW

Sort of Mexican Mole meets North African Tagine, this Spicy Chickpea Stew is incredibly tasty and makes an extraordinary fixing for prepared potatoes, in addition to it simply happens to be veggie lover, vegetarian, gluten free and dairy free. Furthermore, it contains chocolate.

Fixings

- 4-6 preparing potatoes, pricked everywhere

- 2 tablespoons olive oil

- 2 red onions, finely cleaved

- 4 cloves garlic, ground or squashed

- 2cm ginger, ground

- ½ - 2 teaspoons bean stew chips (contingent upon how hot you like things)

- 2 tablespoons cumin seeds

- 2 tablespoons turmeric

- Sprinkle of water

- 2 x 400g tins slashed tomatoes

- 2 tablespoons unsweetened cocoa powder (or cacao)

- 2 x 400g tins chickpeas (or kidney beans on the off chance that you like) including the chickpea water DON'T DRAIN!!

- 2 yellow peppers (or whatever shading you like!), slashed into bite size pieces

- 2 tablespoons parsley in addition to extra for embellish

- Salt and pepper to taste (discretionary)

- Side plate of mixed greens (discretionary)

Strategy

1. Preheat the stove to 200C, in the mean time you can set up the entirety of your fixings.

2. When the stove is hot enough placed your preparing potatoes in the broiler and cook for 1 hour or until they are done how you like them.

3. Once the potatoes are in the broiler, place the olive oil and slashed red onion in an enormous wide pan and cook delicately, with the cover on for 5 minutes, until the onions are delicate however not earthy colored.

4. Remove the top and include the garlic, ginger, cumin and bean stew. Cook for a further moment on a low warmth, at that point include the turmeric and an extremely little sprinkle of water and cook for one more moment, taking consideration not to let the container get excessively dry.

5. Next, include the tomatoes, cocoa powder (or cacao), chickpeas (counting the chickpea water) and yellow pepper. Bring to the bubble,

at that point stew on a low warmth for 45 minutes until the sauce is thick and unctuous (yet don't allow it to consume!). The stew ought to be done at generally a similar time as the potatoes.

6. Finally mix in the 2 tablespoons of parsley, and some salt and pepper on the off chance that you wish, and serve the stew on the prepared potatoes, maybe with a basic side plate of mixed greens.

CONCLUSION

In spite of the fact that the eating regimen is frequently hailed as simple to follow on account of the reality it incorporates red wine and dull chocolate, it's genuinely severe in its rules.

The sirtfood plan depends on health food nuts confining their calorie admission just as eating a particular rundown of nourishments that are said to help the digestion.

An eating routine that stresses dim chocolate, red wine, kale, berries, and espresso? It either seems like the most ideal street to health and weight reduction, or unrealistic. Be that as it may, pause, it shows signs of improvement: According to the makers of the Sirtfood Diet, these and other alleged "sirtfoods" are indicated to enact the systems constrained by your body's characteristic "thin qualities" to assist you with consuming fat and get fit.

Bragging a rundown delicious nourishment, you likely as of now love, and supported by reports that Adele utilized it to shed pounds in the wake of having an infant, the Sirtfood Diet sounds justifiably engaging.

In any case, not to demolish your chocolate-and-red-wine high here, yet the science doesn't really bolster the eating regimen's greatest cases. Which isn't to state that eating sirtfoods is an impractical notion . . . in any case, similarly as with all eating regimens that sound unrealistic, you should take a gander at this one with genuine investigation. This is what you have to think about what sirtfoods can and can't accomplish for you.

Above all else, what the hell is a sirtfood?

Created by U.K. nourishment experts Aidan Goggin's and Glen Matten, the Sirtfood Diet accentuates plant-based food sources that are known "certain activators." Basically, when you nosh on the arrangement's key fixings, you invigorate the proteins encoded for by the SIRT1 quality, which Goggin's and Matten have named "the thin quality."

SIRT1 and certain proteins are accepted to assume a job in maturing and life span, which might be identified with the defensive impacts of calorie limitation. The case behind the Sirtfood Diet is that sure nourishments can actuate these sort-intervened pathways sans the limitation, and in this way "switch on your muscle to fat ratio's consuming forces, supercharge weight reduction, and help fight off malady."

Alongside red wine, dull chocolate, berries, espresso, and kale, certain-advancing nourishments incorporate matcha green tea, additional virgin olive oil, pecans, parsley, red onions, soy, and turmeric (a.k.a. incredible flavors and go-to solid treats).

There's some science behind the cases of sirtfoods' advantages, yet it's exceptionally constrained and rather dubious.

The science on the shirt outskirts is still overly new. There are examines investigating the SIRT1 quality's job in maturing and life span, in maturing related weight increase and maturing related malady, and in shielding the heart from irritation brought about by a high-fat eating routine. However, the exploration is constrained to work done in test tubes and on mice, which is not adequate proof to state that certain-boosting nourishments can have weight reduction or hostile to maturing abilities in a real human body.

Brooke Alpert, R.D., creator of The Sugar Detox, says there's exploration to recommend that the weight-control advantages of sirtfoods may come to a limited extent from the polyphenol-cancer prevention agent resveratrol, frequently advertised as a component in red wine. "All things considered, it is difficult to devour enough red wine to get benefits," she says, taking note of that she does as often as possible recommend resveratrol enhancements to her customers.

Furthermore, some nourishment specialists aren't psyched about the manner in which the Sirtfood Diet plan works.

As per top dietitians who've surveyed the arrangement, the Sirtfood Diet is feeling the loss of some significant components for a solid, adjusted routine. Goggin's and Matten's eating routine arrangement includes three stages: a couple of days at 1,000 calories for each day, comprised of one sirtfood-overwhelming feast and green squeezes; a couple of long stretches of two sirtfood suppers and two squeezes every day, for an aggregate of 1,500 calories; and a fourteen-day support period of shirt-y dinners and juices.

The decision? Sirtfoods are incredible to have in your eating routine, however they shouldn't be all you have.

There's positively no explanation you can't include some sirtfoods into your eating plan, says Alpert. "I think there are some truly fascinating things here, similar to the red wine, dim chocolate, matcha—I love these things," she says. "I love mentioning to individuals what to concentrate on rather than what to nix from their eating routine." If it tastes liberal and it's solid in little amounts, why not?

Be that as it may, all the nourishment specialists propose balancing the eating regimen with some lean protein and sound fats, for example, progressively nuts and seeds, avocado, and greasy fish like salmon. Stir up your plate of mixed greens game, as well, with more kinds of veggies, spinach, and romaine lettuce notwithstanding the kale and red onions. Primary concern? The majority of the sirtfoods are An OK to eat and solid for you, however, simply do not depend on the eating routine to actuate any "thin quality" presently.

Lightning Source UK Ltd.
Milton Keynes UK
UKHW051705130421
381888UK00003BA/334